RUNNING
FROM
CANCER

For Kathy— Aug 1 2013

Wishing you strength,
summer days : good health—

Debi Smith

RUNNING FROM CANCER

a tilted memoir

DebiLyn Smith

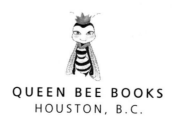

QUEEN BEE BOOKS
HOUSTON, B.C.

ISBN 978-0-9919093-0-8

Queen Bee Books
3001 Gushwa Rd.
Houston, B.C. V0J 1Z1
Canada

Cover design by Ranilo Cabo
Interior design and typesetting by
Williams Writing, Editing & Design
Editing by Lynn Shervill

Lyrics to "Ordinary Day" by Alan Doyle and Sean McCann
of Great Big Sea reprinted with permission.

The information presented in this book is an expression of the author's experiences and intended for informational and educational purposes only — not as a medical instructional manual. This book does not replace professional treatment, and while it offers experiences and wisdom gained by the author, the author in no way is suggesting medical advice or directives. If you are seeking a medical opinion for yourself or your loved one, you are encouraged to see a doctor or other qualified health-care professional to make informed and balanced choices.

Anecdotes from the author's life, although based on real incidents, contain situations where some names (including all physician's initials) have been changed to protect the privacy of the individuals.

There are link addresses to websites which are not under the control of the author or publisher. We have no control over the nature, content and availability of those sites. The inclusion of any links does not necessarily imply a recommendation or endorse the views expressed within them.

For Mom who gracefully led the way
For my brother who did it his way
And for my sister who was there for us all

Contents

Preface

You can run, but you can't hide. Like everything else in my life, I found this out the hard way. When it comes to cancer there are no rules and nothing is fair. It's a nasty ordeal. The therapy used to battle the disease can be just as nasty. I can attest to the saying "they have to just about kill you before they cure you" as being quite accurate.

Enduring the process is much easier when you know what lies ahead. Half of my anxiety and nervousness was due to lack of knowledge. I knew nothing about cancer. Until I got the disease, life was busy with no health-oriented focus or goals. Then I lost half a breast and gained a few scars. The positive news is I now weigh less, have thicker post-chemo hair and, best of all, have developed a killer attitude on how to stop running from cancer. Now I stand firm and fight back.

I fell into the cancer sea as a Surface Girl, mere flotsam on the water refusing to get in too deep . . . until the diagnosis of breast cancer threatened to sink me. I came out a virtual cancer lifeguard, eager to aid others to stay afloat.

Like pregnancy texts that never admit childbirth is painful, the cancer texts never say with clarity what breast surgery, chemotherapy and radiation are really like in terms of what you feel before, during and after. It's not a picnic but it is certainly doable. Knowing more about the experience from a survivor's side can help you or someone you love take steps to prevent cancer or to deal effectively with the disease once it's diagnosed. That's why I wrote this book.

I didn't go down this road easily. I was a 50-year-old freelance writer, my best asset being my Attention Deficit Disorder (ADD), which gave me an unlimited supply of imagination, impulsivity and energy. It also burdened me with endless trepidation, indecision and a strong desire to run away screaming from anything scary.

Being diagnosed with any type of cancer is a life-altering moment. If you catch it in time to do something about it, your existence will still morph into a world of appointments and waiting rooms, needles and tests, surgeries and drugs. I was dragged down further than I ever thought possible but it was all for a reason. It was my wake-up call. I couldn't change the verdict but I could darn well do something to prevent a recurrence. Having cancer is devastating but it can also save your life. It's all about attitude. My glass is half full and I thank cancer for redeeming me from myself and my self-destructive habits. Turns out, my worst enemy was me.

At the beginning of 2008 the word cancer was nothing but another type of cootie: a folklore disease I feared catching as a child. I didn't know exactly what cancer was but I knew I didn't want to get it. I couldn't see it on anybody walking around. I couldn't even tell who had it or who didn't. I never considered it might touch my life. My family was healthy. Cancer was something that happened to others.

It wasn't like I turned a blind eye. I ran for the Cure. I bought daffodils for the Cure. But I didn't personally know anyone that needed the Cure.

All that was about to change.

Life is full of ups and downs. We enjoy the rise more than the fall, yet what would life be without the triumph of struggle, the standing, feet firmly planted with hands on hips, to face your terrors? The answer is life would be wonderful! But it wouldn't be real. Getting cancer these days is not so much an "if" as it is a "when."

There is a painting on my desk that simply says "Hope." It was made by a 12-year-old wanting to give a gift of the word to someone who might need it. I love that painting because it epitomizes what having cancer is all about: the part where you look in the mirror and say, "I will do what I can to beat cancer."

The earlier you start fighting cancer, the more hope you have.

Right now would be a good time.

1

Sizing Up Cancer

My initiation into the world of cancer began in July 2008 with my husband Barry's sweet Aunt Joleen. Terminal with colon cancer, her existence was as fragile as her bones, which could break with the slightest stress. Barry and I raced to visit her while she was still able to sit on the porch with us and enjoy a beer.

Squinting in the sun, Jo took a sip from her can, the foam leaving a slight white line above her chapped upper lip. Her smile was intact but inky shadows haunted the under part of her eyes. Her billowy blouse rarely connected to a contour, like a sheet hanging on a clothesline.

"It was nice of you kids to stop in. That was a long drive from up north. On your way to Vancouver, are you?"

My husband squirmed in his chair. "No, just thought we'd come to see you, Aunt Jo."

Joleen tucked a misplaced lock of wavy hair behind her ear. She looked down at the faded, synthetic slippers on her feet before lifting her head, a wide grin on her thin face.

"All that way to visit Bob and me? Well, isn't that a nice thing to have done." She took another small sip of her beer. "You didn't have to do that. But I'm glad you did. So tell me, what's new in your lives?"

She leaned back, deep into the lounge chair she was propped up in. A shadow of pain crossed her profile, her deeply veined fingers clenched for a long second before she let out her breath with a sigh. She looked back at us expectantly. *Distract me, please.*

Barry grabbed for his drink, determined to keep busy with it. It had been my idea we come. He wanted to be here but he didn't. It was eating him up, I could see.

"Everything is great," I told her. "The kids are all happy with their lives, Barry is enjoying his semi-retirement and I'm still writing. But how about you? Are they able to control the pain, Jo?"

"What happened to your leg?" she asked, pointing at my scabbed and bruised left shin.

A change of subject. There would be no questions about her health.

"That? That is compliments of our neighbour's dog, Banner." I rubbed my finger over the tender area. "He chases me when I jog by. I tripped this time and wiped out on the rocks. Thankfully he'd already given up the game."

No one else said anything so I blathered on. "There's no other way past. I almost hate to go running. He's making my life a living hell."

A sharp barking noise made us both look up from my leg to Joleen. She was laughing.

She gently slapped one emaciated knee. "A dog," she repeated, her eyes full of merriment. "I'd forgotten what it must feel like to be chased." She coughed as she tried to let another laugh slip out. "Let's hope, my dear, that's as bad as it gets for you."

Still smiling, Joleen struggled to stand, quickly helped by her husband's hand. "I need a nap," she said, kissing us and hugging as best as her remaining strength allowed. "Thanks so much for coming."

She turned and looked right at me. "You're such a kicker," she said, her grin once more filling her face. "Thanks."

Joleen died weeks later, and I realized she was the first person with cancer I had spoken to, kissed, hugged, and bade goodbye as if she were soon off on an exotic holiday. I'd like to think that's what happened.

I decided after the tragedy of Joleen that I could become a little more proactive about my own life. Now 48, I had two children, had been divorced and remarried, and was just 20 pounds overweight. I joked that the ring around my waist, comprised of dry martinis, red wines, chocolate truffles and countless sushi rolls cost my second husband more than the new ring around my finger. What a riot.

I went to the gym three times a week to socialize with my gal pals, lift a few weights and gab while strolling on the treadmill. Able to outrun everyone I knew but Banner, I figured I was the picture of safe health, a walking commercial for women my age.

In my dreams.

I ate packaged sauces, double cream desserts and soft, doughy white bread, thinking nothing of it until I had two mini strokes (called Transient Ischemic Attacks or TIAs) in November, one right- and one left-brained within hours of each other. Same as with Aunt Jo's cancer, the experience should have been a real eye-opener. Like in the movie *Sixth Sense*, this was my first red doorknob, the fore-shadowing of things to come. But I missed it. I still did not under-stand that life could and would go sideways when you least expected it, that good health wasn't a gimme.

After a CT (computerized tomography) and MRI (magnetic res-onance imaging) scan, the stroke specialist said this might have hap-pened from the stress of working three jobs. He told me to unwind and suggested I lose the spare-tire waist before it ran me over. He swore my ADD medication, Ritalin, could not be the culprit for the TIAs but took me off it anyway. He was right to do so. Two years later, after a young boy's death made headline news, Ritalin came with the warning "may cause strokes." The pills constricted blood vessels through which I'd been piping blobs of deep-fried chicken skin and high-fat cream cheese.

That's my perception of the situation, medically correct or not. Bottom line . . . I had looked death in the face and not known it.

So, what did I do? I shrugged my shoulders. I was not at the stage yet where I would realize the gift I had been given, the signal to change course. Life went back to normal.

I was put on a new drug to lower my cholesterol, which I figured gave me back the license to eat poorly whenever I felt like it. Okay, maybe I used a little less gravy on my mashed potatoes and switched from full-fat sour cream and mayonnaise to light, but that was the extent of the compromise. There was always that premenstrual demand to break out the community-sized bag of potato chips or consume my body weight in chocolate.

Marginally back on track, my health appeared perfect again. I did start to talk less and exercise more at the gym, hoping to wake up to an image that fit inside my mirror.

My husband's left eyebrow shot up at the mounded second plate of lasagna I had dished myself.

"Still hungry?" he asked.

"Yeh, I worked really hard at the gym this morning. A circuit training class, then we went running for twenty." My fork went into automated scoop-and-shovel mode.

"Okay," he drew the word out slowly like he was testing what he was going to say in his head first, "and you're trying to lose how much weight?"

The fork stopped mid-air. *Where was this going?*

"There's no number. I'm just trying to lose a bit."

"How much weight?"

Okay. Fine. Dream weight of 145 pounds for my 5 feet 7 inches frame. "Eighteen to go."

Barry stood and came around to where I sat, fork still hanging mid-air with a clump of glistening high-fat cheese oozing down.

We both looked at it. I put my fork down.

Once I stomped away from the table, I noticed I wasn't hungry anymore. My meal had caught up with my brain.

Okay, so Barry was right. It all came down to calories in versus calories out. Bolstered with enthusiasm, I decided I would hold the chocolate sauce and whipped cream on my dessert. I smiled at myself. What a trooper. I was headed in the right direction.

It would have been easier if three of my grandparents hadn't passed prematurely — one in WWII and two in a tragic car accident when they were in their early 50s. It eliminated my crystal ball of probability. . . messages like "You better watch your cholesterol levels. Grandpa dropped after a bucket of fried chicken just like that one."

My maternal grandmother died from lung cancer, but we put that down to the two-pack-a-day habit and never gave cancer another thought. I told my doctor that cancer didn't run in my family. I wonder how long he shook his head after I left.

Everyone has the ability to make cancer cells. They are just normal cells that go haywire and refuse to die when they're supposed to. Like little forest fires, they get bigger and start to grow. Your body is continually stamping those fires out. If you have a strong immune system, no problem; it could kick cancer's butt all day long and keep winning the fight. But if you're not fueling your body with the right fire retardant, then the blaze can get out of control. Cancer cells divide at a much faster rate than normal cells, so the fire intensifies, overwhelming your defences.

Scientists aren't sure what exactly kick-starts a cancer cell into dividing, multiplying and taking over but you can decrease the risk. Don't smoke. Avoid junk food. Be active. But in 2008, I was pretty sure I wouldn't get it. I lived a fairly risk-free life. I washed my hands faithfully after every visit to the washroom. I ate lots of vegetables and ordered whole wheat buns at the fast-food joints. Why would I need to prevent something I was sure I wouldn't get?

To be on the safe side though, I read the health articles in my women's magazines about skin, breast and cervical cancers, something I usually skipped over as they did not pertain to me. On their advisement I started putting blueberries and flax seed in my oatmeal every morning. It took me awhile to realize the flax seeds had to be freshly ground to be effective, but I got there eventually.

The articles talked about sugar and nutritionally empty foods like white rice, white pasta and white breads that broke down into sugar. Worse, when you consumed refined sugar it made you crave more sugar, and sugar is an enemy. Cancer cells thrive on sugar and excess fat, meaning that extra stuff you may be packing on your belly, thighs and butt. It's a super simplistic way of putting it, but the end result was I had an addiction to things that could make me more miserable than I could ever dream possible. Still, I figured I would lose weight on my terms in my own time. It's behaviour typical of a Surface Girl.

I had quit smoking years ago so I figured I was safe there. I drank more alcohol than was recommended, but I didn't have a problem with alcohol. Like my friends, I enjoyed a glass of wine most nights with dinner, slipping past two glasses to more like a bottle all to myself on weekend evenings. I sipped a glass while prepping dinner, had a glass with my meal, one after cleanup and a glass while playing cards or chatting for three more hours. That was at least a bottle of wine. Not the healthiest thing to do, but what could it hurt? It was red wine. Wasn't that good for you and your vascular system? I was still hiking, skiing, swimming or bicycling to keep my body fat in check. I had begun jogging and doing sit-ups with my friends. I thought I was a bouncing commercial for a vital 40s lifestyle. Now that I'm awake, I see there was a noose around my neck that was slowly tightening.

The next phase of my cancer journey, after Joleen, began with my mother. I knew Mom wouldn't live forever. The natural progression of life is your pet dies, your grandparents die, your parents die, then you die. When I was 10, I thought the world had ended with my hamster's burial.

"But what happened to Yogi, Mom?" He didn't look like he was sleeping. His eyes were all bugged out and his fur was wet. "Is that what Grandpa looked like when he died?"

"No, no," Mom said, helping me up from beside the wooden cross inscribed with the words R.I.P. Yogi. Dirty tears rolled down my face and my mother licked her fingertips and stroked my cheek clean.

"Grandpa just went to sleep and didn't wake up. I think possibly Yogi wasn't well. Maybe he was sick when we bought him."

This made me cry harder. *Had he been in pain all that time?*

"Nobody lives forever, Deb," she tried.

I looked up at her, the idea of what she said sinking further and further in until I was attending the funerals of my mother, father, brother and sister in my head.

They were all going to die!

"No," I moaned as I pulled my arm out of my mother's grasp and fled to my bedroom. It was all too horrible to think about. I threw myself onto my unmade bed, my gaze resting on the empty hamster cage on my desk. I cried until my sister Kim arrived with a bag of Oreos.

"You can play with one of my Barbie dolls," she said, and all was right with the world again.

I was too young to remember the tragedy of my grandparents' motor vehicle accident and too far away to be there for my maternal grandmother's passing. I made it to her funeral and shed more tears that day for my mother than for her mother. I realized the sadness stayed with those left behind. They were the ones who needed the sympathy, not the dearly departed. Like everything else, experiencing the death of a loved one has a learning curve. I was merely in grade school at this point.

The earth moves. It struggles and grinds and shoves up pieces of itself to create new lands where none once existed. I wasn't waiting for anything so impressive to happen in my life. I wanted only for Banner, the neighbour's dog, to die. To be hit by a car, to choke on a bone, to be shot by someone else terrorized by its charging with teeth bared and hackles raised. Anything to break the vicious cycle of warding off the dog every time I went for a run. I phoned the owners but they said to try throwing a stick for it to chase. I tried that. The stick bounced off Banner's head, guaranteeing the chase would continue with a vengeance for the rest of our days together.

Time and the chases dragged on. Other neighbours commiserated with me about the dog as it raced after anything that moved. There were all sorts of spectacular suggestions, none of them realistic. There was but one answer. We would have to outlive it. Dogs last what, 15 years tops? It had already been five. It was only a glimmer, but there was hope. If you don't like what's happening, just wait.

Things do change.

February 2009

Dear Deb . . .

You would not believe how many of my friends are sick with the flu.

I am fine. The stomach/pancreas test I had today said I have nothing wrong and should not need antacids. However, the specialist couldn't answer my question of why then, the pain I have been having for over a month.

Hmm. The specialist said my doctor won't get the report for over a week and my doctor will be gone then for two weeks. Great. So, then if he wanted another test I will wait some more. Damn. Ah well, it could be something really bad and I am sure this is obviously not bad. Just a ruddy pain in the neck.

Geesh!

Love,
Ma xoxo

———————

Then it happened. The dog that terrorized me every morning for years was gone. In the blink of an eye, the space of a weekend, Banner had chased the wrong car. I remember thinking what a good day it was. I had waited for it and the inevitable had happened.

After my run I took a shower, made some lunch and treated myself to a celebratory glass of Sauvignon Blanc. A wee toast to the end of my dog troubles.

The phone rang. I waved my wine glass toward the sound. "Cheers to the phone." I looked at the wall clock: 2 p.m.

"Hello?"

Funny how one minute you're breathing and the next you're not.

"Did I catch you busy?" Mom always started a conversation this way, as if something might be more important than hearing from her.

"Hi ya, Ma. No, I finished eating and Barry's at the drugstore. They were short a pharmacist so he's filling in for the week. What's up?"

And yes, I talk like that. It's an ADD bottom-line thing. The pleasantries of conversation like asking people how they are or how their day went always came after I knew what the call was about. I wish now I'd remembered that about myself.

"Okay. Well, I, uhm . . ."

I hooked the phone between my chin and shoulder and set about stacking my plate and bowl from the table. I wondered if it was snowing where she lived. I hadn't been paying my usual attention to her weather in New Brunswick, which differed greatly from ours 5000 miles away in British Columbia.

Mom's voice came out quieter than usual. I could barely hear what she said next. Something about tests returning and what was that?

"Pancreatic cancer," she said a little louder. "Stage IVB. They said it has spread to my liver. That's not good."

I'm not usually speechless. The silverware in my hand crashed to the table as I reached up to grab the phone from my neck.

"Mom, you have cancer?" The words froze in my throat as the

warmth ran from my body. I had no idea what to add to that. I was flabbergasted. Gob-smacked. Lasered from outer space. Whatever was she talking about?

"It's true, dear. I'm so sorry."

She was sorry?

"I've told Kim and now I have to call your brother next."

"But are you okay? Did they say how long you have? Are you in pain?" Now the questions flooded in. Where was an airplane? Maybe I should grab a bag, start running and hope the airplane would catch up to me? I'm coming, Mom, I'm coming.

One year, possibly less.

And because this isn't a fairy tale, it would end up being much less.

Mom and I didn't talk long; she wanted to call my brother Danny, who also lived in British Columbia, a mere 14-hour drive south of us. Danny was married and had two teenagers. Mom wanted to reach him before the kids got home from school.

I stumbled downstairs to the computer and searched frantically for information but the more I read on her condition the more I screamed out to the empty room. My mother was going to die a painful death from a cancer so far advanced there was no stopping it.

I wanted to go home. Right now! My parents were divorced years earlier and Dad had since remarried. Mom was there all alone. OMG, OMG, OMG. This could not be happening. She was as trim and slim and fit as a fiddle. How could this woman get cancer? What had gone wrong?

Other than the short experience with Aunt Joleen, the C-word was still somewhere out there, beyond my periphery. I was a spoiled, protected 49-year-old busy trying to ward off *big* things like grey hair, wrinkled cleavage and a dog that loved to make me wet my pants.

On March 10 I got a letter from my sister, who had flown in to be with Mom.

Hi!

As you know, Mom went to the hospital for pain management and ended up being admitted; just until they can get the pain under control enough that she can self-administer her medication at home.

We had a great Saturday. Mom was quite chipper and rearranged her hospital room a few times. She walked down to the nurses' station and the family room, which was the furthest she has ventured in a few days. I was sent off for a walk and came back to Mom entertaining again. She was good and kept her feet up to help reduce the swelling in her legs. I started giving her a big cup of ice water with a straw, and refilled it about six times, which is great because her mouth becomes really dry. She has also become quite attached to my Chap Stick I gave her. Ha. She had me bring in my laptop with some computer files from Rotary to finish up, which made her feel quite good (she said so a few times!). She enjoyed talking with Danny's family in the morning and Deb when she called.

She is learning to ask for pain medication and not wait until the next dose (she was trying to hold on). The nurse Tracey was really good and told Mom she was only here because Mom was here, so if Mom did not call her, what was Tracey to do? She reminded Mom that unless Mom helped them, it would be longer before she got to go home.

After all the activity, Mom ended the day with a very sore lower back (this is mainly the pancreas, they tell me). They gave her an extra 5 mg of Oxi IR for the breakthrough (as they call the in-between dosages) and her usual 10 mg which she gets every four hours (2-6-10-2-6-10). She also gets a blood thinner and a combined stool softener/laxative. Her legs and feet are still swollen from all the fluid (which they say is from low protein, low sodium levels and from the disease). She takes an antibiotic, as her left ankle got some infection from blistering due to the swelling. She had another 500 ml bag of sodium to bring her up to normal, and we're going to retest her blood Sunday a.m. to make sure it is okay.

Mom still gets really tired quite easily (says she is weary) and this can make it so she mumbles and it is hard to understand her, but when she is not tired it can seem like we are sitting gabbing in her living room. She is very thin (yes, even thinner than usual) and her cheeks have become quite gaunt. But she has this tummy that we joke makes her look about four or five months pregnant! This is from the disease, her fluid retention and the low sodium.

We end each day with the two of us picking up, throwing out, putting everything in order — things like pillows and cups seem to accumulate. I take back the dirty PJs and have brought a stash of clean ones (T-shirts and fleece bottoms). I have been leaving around eight or so (it was 9:30 last night) and getting there around eight in the morning when she wakes up and breakfast comes.

This morning (Sunday), I have been told to go to church to see her pastor Father W. again. I should be at the hospital around 11 if you want to call.

Love you all,

Kim

On March 18, I fret through all three flights to get us — Barry and me — from Smithers to Vancouver, Vancouver to Toronto and Toronto to Fredericton. That was a lot of ups and downs. What if a flight was delayed? Could we still make our connections? What if we experienced plane or weather problems? Mom said this wasn't going to be an instant keel over, but still I worried. Would we make it before she left us?

My first instinct was to self-medicate, but I hadn't hugged Mom in over a year and didn't want her to smell booze on my breath. Had it really been 15 months since the last time we were in the same room together? That might sound bad, but the truth is Mom and I were not as close as she was with Danny and Kim. I'd read a lot of books on the subject, trying to understand how a two-month-old could rebel against her mother the way I was told I did. That reading led to the realization my parents were not perfect.

They had married in Ontario in 1957 — a tire salesman and a junior accountant — before moving to the smaller province of New Brunswick, a good 24-hour drive away. Danny was born the day after their first wedding anniversary and within a year Dorothy was pregnant again with me.

That didn't mean everything was roses.

They say ADD is hereditary and I don't have to look far for the source of my affliction. My father is an ADD poster child. It's one of the few attributes, besides my crooked nose, that proved, un-equivocally, my connection to this family even though my brother swore I was adopted.

A young and handsome man, Dad had the attention span of a yo-yo and didn't acknowledge that actions had consequences until it was too late. As I mentioned, people with ADD tend to learn everything the hard way, although we do have a great time as it happens. It takes a lot to harness us.

He still won't say why Mom grabbed her infant son and her maternity clothes that year and moved back to Ontario to live with her parents.

I was born on a stormy, winter night in London, Ontario. My grandmother's car got stuck in a snow bank and my labouring mother had to hail a cab to get to the hospital. My birthing was long and troublesome. I didn't like to be forced to do anything, even back then. It's no wonder Mom spiraled down into a deep postpartum depression. The new baby girl would have to wait to have a mother who could cope with her.

In the meantime, I was plugged into bottles and propped up with blankets instead of being held in my mother's arms. It's the only thing I can think of as to why the bond between us was always strained. She never recovered from thinking of me as the baby she conceived while her blissful marriage was a lie. I was an icon of deceit.

"Oh, don't flatter yourself," my sister says. "You're not always the centre of everything."

Admittedly I was the devil's spawn at times. From the get-go I wouldn't eat what everyone else ate. I think I was the only kid in the world who wanted to send my hot dogs and apple pie to the starving children in Africa. I was an inquisitive, noisy top always spinning out of control. My father said children like me were often found abandoned. He wasn't smiling.

It was a week after I was born that Dad came to see his new baby and try to collect his family. Whatever he said worked and we all returned to New Brunswick. My beautiful sister Kim arrived 18 months later.

All this raced through my mind as I punched at the hospital's elevator buttons a half dozen times. Was she still with us? Did I miss my chance to say goodbye, to say I was sorry for every little and every big thing I might have done to annoy her? It was a long list. I would need lots of time.

I stopped at the nurses' station for information and got steered toward the palliative care unit. *Palliative care? Already?*

Mom was only in the hospital to try and get her pain under control! Something must have changed.

Her room was the second door down on the right. I took a large breath and straightened my travel outfit of wrinkled skirt and even crinklier jacket. I readjusted my smile, patted down my rooster tail and imagined the cheeriest thoughts I could.

Ready, I walked in, immediately alarmed by her appearance. I tried hard to hold it back but my eyes popped wider and my smile slipped at the sight of black sores encrusting her entire upper lip, at how thin she was, at how tired she looked, at the first sight of grey in her sporty blonde hair. I had never before thought of her as old but there it was right in front of me. It was a big shock. I had been shocked before, but it never felt like this. This was almost a feeling of betrayal. When had she become so aged? This was the single mom who still skied and kayaked and rode her bike for hours, the woman who lived on the third floor of a lift-less apartment building — who, as the building's superintendent, dragged a 10-pound vacuum cleaner up and down the steps once a week. Where did that Mom go?

She had fooled us, fooled us all, and she would be so pleased to hear me tell it that way. The expensive spot-softening and wrinkle-defying creams and all the hats she used to protect her face from the sun's damaging rays had paid off. The friends who never ceased arriving and hugging and saying goodbye to her all thought she was much younger than she was. To the end, Mother would not tell them — and forbade us to tell them — her actual age. Her obituary had already been written and given to the funeral home and it did not state the year she was born.

No wonder I was as confused as the rest. Only I had no excuse. I knew what year she was born and exactly what age she was. I just never thought of her as old enough to die, not someone as healthy and alive as she was.

You couldn't see Mom once I folded myself around her. For all my strength and resolve, the sobs still managed to slip from my throat. I couldn't let her go. I clung harder, not realizing my thick winter coat was smothering her. She slugged my arm and pushed me backward, but with tenderness and a smile. "What are you doing," she asked, "trying to kill me?

"No tears," she demanded, rubbing my arm but still giving me The Look.

"Okay, yep. I love you, Mom. I love you so much."

"I know. I love you too. I'm so glad you both came."

She gestured for Barry and me to take a seat on a little couch inside her room. We drank tea and tried to feel like we were anywhere but in a hospital. My brother and his wife arrived from the airport. There were smiles and laughs, memories and slight confessions, one concerning a bottle of vodka that had gone missing when the three kids were teens.

The following week was a blur of organizing Mom's last birthday party. It was held in the palliative care unit's family room with all her friends in attendance. They brought pot luck and we took pictures. There were gifts of chocolates and flowers and poems and books. We put together a PowerPoint picture presentation of Mom's life. Her story played out before her eyes. She'd had an amazing run.

The day exhausted her but she remained stoic, classy to the end. She was able to find the energy to quip a sharp "Deb, cut it out," when my feelings got the better of me and I was pouting, feeling left out of her entourage.

It was an emotionally draining time, especially when Barry had to return to B.C. for work. I stayed behind, intending to join him in time for a vacation we'd scheduled. We said our goodbyes after the birthday party.

My sister, who works for the government, was between jobs, ending one and being interviewed for another. She had to return to Ottawa but was determined to come back before Mom got much worse. Kim only needed a few days. I insisted she go, assuring her Mom and I would be fine.

This worked well for me as Kim really wanted to be with Mom when she passed. I have to confess the notion terrified me. I had never seen anyone die before and was wary of what I might do. Or say. Okay, I was a big, fat coward who didn't want to face the reality of it all. I wanted to say my tearful goodbyes to my mother and be off on the trip through the Panama Canal that Barry and I had booked with friends a year prior. I would have to mourn Mom's passing as best I could from there and that felt fine with me. Callous but true. My sister would be with Mom until the end. It's what Mom wanted. It's what Kim wanted. And I was okay with it. Danny was okay with it. So it was settled.

Don't get me wrong. I loved my mother very much. Over the years, especially after having my own children, I began to appreciate her in my life. Our friendship strengthened and blossomed. Still, I remained doubtful of how good a daughter I had been until I was presented with a hefty bag holding every single card I had sent to my mother over 40-plus years.

"You saved these all this time?" I asked, incredulous and not without some guilt for not having done the same for my own children. I rummaged through the stack, recognizing some, not recognizing even more. I flipped them all open and there were my words for her. Love lined the pages, my admiration unmistakable.

"I kept everything," she told me. "I thought maybe you could use it one day. There's great humour in there."

My number one fan 'til the end. She had bought me my first typewriter for Christmas when I was 10. It was tan-coloured plastic with a blurry, blue ribbon, but it worked well enough for me and my stories.

Despite all of that, I still say it's not everyone that can sit and hold a parent's hand while they die. And if my sister wanted that job and Mom was fine with it, then so was I. Yes, I had a big fat yellow stripe down my back, a walking, talking commercial for cowardice.

The plan was accepted. Kim flew to Ontario to get her life into a more suitable holding pattern. She would return to Mom's side and spend as long as was warranted. Danny and his wife returned to Invermere to their own hectic business.

Mother and I carried on at the hospital. Her schedule included bandage changes for the infected sore on her ankle, a daily trek to the shower down the hall, three meals a day, constant creaming of her lips, her puffy tight skin and her cracked, purplish feet and always, always keeping our outer cheer up. The stream of friends, nurses, doctors and other caregivers kept us scrambling. I was exhausted just trying to keep up to it all.

There's a recurring theme in my life, the part where I think I have things under control.

The reins were in my hands but I was so busy trying to match my sister's recent endurance and thoughtfulness I hadn't noticed Mom's downward spiral. There was more writhing in-between her medication shots, more "breakthrough" pain, as the hospital staff called it. The trips to the shower ended as it was "too far to go to the end of the hall." She quit eating. Her meals started to arrive pureed, but she never wanted to try any of it. She stuck to water and juice only because I nattered at her. Visitors were turned away because she slept most of the time. I watched her snore with great racking attempts to get in more oxygen.

Journal Entry
April 2, 2009

I feel so stupid, so caught napping while life crashed around me. Am I the only one left who doesn't have a clue about cancer? I know nothing. Or is that true? Grandma died from lung cancer ages ago. She walked around her last year with an oxygen tank tucked under her arm like it was a cocktail purse. The smoke from her straw-length cigarette swirled around her free hand while the other held onto the rubber tubing that went from her nostrils to the tank-of-life, now a permanent metal fixture near her body. Gram was a walking advertisement for quitting smoking, a tree made only of bark, the wood inside long ago rotted away by the cancer.

I know about the colour of cancer. I watched as it bubbled and frothed from my mother's lips yesterday, her eyes wild in wonder at what was happening inside of her. It was filth, blackened coffee grounds that stank of hell. It was disease coming to the surface,

*poking evil tentacles at the people bending sore backs over the shell
that was once a vital and spirited figure.*

*I know that I hate cancer. I want it to die. But that would mean
willing Mom to die as well. Yet, looking at her now, I don't think she
wants to stay here anymore. Her dreams of being elsewhere take her
away longer every day.*

Two days later the nurses suggested I move into Mom's room.

"What? What for?" I asked, my eyes wide in terror.

Okay, I knew what for. I just wasn't ready to be there for the
"what for."

"Already? Are we at that stage, are you sure? It's only been two
months?"

This couldn't be happening. My sister wasn't due back for another three days.

I phoned Mom's priest. He arrived and I mumbled her last prayer
for her while she nodded and received her blessing. I phoned my
sister, who was on the road between Ottawa and Toronto, and held
the phone to Mom's ear, prompting her to say goodbye. Mom managed the single word, "Bye." You could see how taxing it was and that
she was spent with the effort. I phoned my brother and although
Mom had her eyes closed and never spoke again, I knew she was
listening and heard every word Danny had to say.

It was after 10 that night when Kim phoned to say someone had
missed their flight on the overbooked plane. She had a seat on the
last flight of the evening out of Toronto. The entire waiting room
had erupted in applause when her tearful standby status changed
and the flight started to board. It was a miracle. Could I get someone
to pick her up at the Fredericton airport in two hours? I made an
emotional call to one of Mom's best friends, who jumped from her
warm bed and drove the 40 minutes to the airport to rescue my sister.

Angels were flying everywhere overhead.

Together, Kim and I stood, looking down at our mother, watching as she took her last morphine-laced breath. Her eyelids flashed open, and for a moment Mom looked like she was seeing the most amazing sight of her life. She smiled, arched her back ever so slightly. And she was gone.

We were holding her hands, one on either side. I was sounding like a cheerleader, repeating, "Go, Mom, go! Go, Mom, go," waving her onto a plane without pain, without worry and unfortunately, without us.

I left a few days later on my scheduled holiday, hoping I wouldn't have to look into the face of cancer again for a while. Sadly, that while would last a mere 15 months.

2

The Troublesome Pea

Between us, Barry and I have four children from our previous marriages. Barry's oldest is Kelly, born in June; my oldest is Karly, also born in June. Notice that both names start with a *K*? Barry's youngest, Lindsay, born in August, graduated from university with the same degree as my youngest, Lorne, also born in August. Notice that Lindsay and Lorne both start with *L*s?

If you're into astrology, you might find it uncanny that besides our children, Barry's mother and mine are both Aries and our dads are born on cusps. Yet my husband and I, a Gemini and a Sagittarian, are complete polar opposites, June and December. The books say we will either hate each other or be a ying to the other's yang.

Depending on the hour, it could go either way in our house. (Yeh? Well yang you too!)

Being total contraries, he sees something one way and I another. That can work if you're filling out a crossword puzzle together. For the rest of it, he prefers brown and blue to my rainbows, chunky potato salad to my whipped one, Johnny Horton to my Nickelback. The bottom line is we can't fold a blanket together, never mind agree the blanket needs to be folded.

They say opposites attract, and we do find it hard to keep our hands to ourselves. Even when we sleep, one part of us is always touching the other. He is very handsome, from the straight Roman nose and deep-set brown eyes right down to the warm, flat feet.

What they don't tell you is that opposites both attract and repel. I yearn to be more organized and sensible like him; he is drawn to my joie de vivre. He hates my chaos. I hate his penchant for order. After 20-some years, though, we're getting the hang of it. We've learned to communicate. Sort of.

"Hi, I'm home."

"Great. Did you get the water container refilled?"

"What water container?"

"The five gallon one I buckled into the passenger seat of the Suburban."

"Oh that. I thought it was a joke. Why didn't you just ask me to get some water?"

"I thought it was obvious. The empty container is seated beside you and it needs to be filled."

"It's not *obvious*. Besides, there is another full container in the house."

"No, it's not full anymore. I made soup and groats and it's almost empty again. Why couldn't you have just got some water?"

"Because as I said, I didn't think we needed any. Why didn't you just ask me to get some?"

"Because as I told you, I thought it was obvious . . ." and around it goes.

Depending on the day, I could have been the person who needed the water or the person who didn't get any. We bicker incessantly, but as they say, no fight means no making up. Obviously something is there for us to willingly continue beating our heads against a wall 24/7.

Sadly, Kelly and Lindsay had to deal with their mother's passing due to lung cancer in 2000. I thought about how crappy it would be for them if their stepmom was to go down the same path. Never mind what it would do to Barry and my two children. Watching a rerun of my mother's ordeal was something I wouldn't wish on anyone. It was time to shape up. Cancer now *did* run in my family, and I was determined to outrun it.

Typical of anyone with ADD, I plunged headfirst into the world of cancer, going in three directions at once. I gathered stacks of books and magazines, anything that talked about awareness or prevention. I watched doctor shows on TV and sifted through a million articles on the Internet about what vitamins to take, what to avoid, what to embrace. Go vegan, no dairy, no gluten, no sugar, no cooking. Eat everything raw. Drink only natural spring water and use vinegar and baking soda to clean everything, including your oven, teeth and hair. Don't breathe the polluted air or use bleached paper products. Skip the hair dye and if it isn't organic don't put it in your mouth without soaking it in a cleanser (vinegar and baking soda) for 30 minutes first.

There were tales of holistic healing, ravings over miracle pills and medical advice from sites with minimal credentials. Snake oil, shark fin soup, bee pollen, cannabis cream — plenty of information. It was a lengthy passing train and I wondered, *Where to board?* There didn't seem to be a beginning or an end. And there were no guarantees any of it would work.

I was an easy mark, like someone shopping for groceries when hungry. Except I was shopping for vitamins and immune-system boosters while running from the cancer cooties.

Never did I stop to think that you don't "get" cancer; it's not from sitting on the wrong toilet seat or beside someone with weird spots.

Still, I sifted out a list of things with which to arm myself against cancer. I bumped up the leafy green vegetables in my meals, ate more wild salmon and chicken than red meat, popped vitamin D supplements and drank green tea. I ate even *more* blueberries and flax seeds with my oatmeal every morning and tried to cut down on the sugar intake. I breathed easier, thinking I was safe. It was like hiding under my bed with my eyes closed. If I couldn't see the monster, it wasn't there.

I did not slow down with the drinking. The week consisted of planning meals and shopping from Monday to Wednesday before heading up to our ski cabin on Hudson Bay Mountain. There we packed our water, food, clothes and alcohol up through the deep snow to our log abode, warmed ourselves by the fireplace and sipped Grand Marnier and amaretto-laced "blueberry teas" before meeting friends in the ski hill lounge. Over the next four days we would both imbibe merrily with no holding back.

I figured my vitamin regime would ensure disease never caught up to me. Alcohol couldn't hurt me, could it? Grapes were good for you! Talk about clueless.

It's here that I will introduce a big player in my life, a best friend named Sandi. Sandi is a doctor who had a general practice in Houston. She sold the practice years ago and works mainly weekends in emergency at the hospital in the neighbouring town of Smithers. On Tuesdays and Thursdays, she runs a "female clinic" at our Houston Health Centre doing breast and pelvic exams. We jokingly call her our B&B — or boob and bush — doctor. She looks after *only* those areas. Women see their family doctor for other medical needs.

Sandi is a very busy, younger woman, my junior by five years. I remind her of that whenever we're jogging uphill. Sandi is also my fitness, ski and hiking partner. She knows firsthand what shape I'm in and these days, it's great. I have shed excess pounds, and I'm beginning to think I will achieve my weight goal. My clothes fit perfectly because I observe the calories-in versus calories-out thing. If I want cake for dessert, I get off my butt and walk around the block for 40 minutes. Not into exercise today? That's fine, but no high fat cheese or bread for 24 hours. It seemed to be working.

When Sandi heard of my cancer concerns she told me that colon cancer was one of the top three most common causes of cancer

death in the U.S., Canada, and Europe. Next to lung cancer it was
also the most preventable cause of cancer death, thanks to occult
blood tests (blood in the stool) and colonoscopies.

There's a Health Canada commercial on television that advises
you to book a colonoscopy if you're 50 or over. It made sense to
me, like checking the ends of a melon to see if it was rotten anywhere. Probably a good idea after all I'd put myself through the past
35 years. We're talking tons of processed mac and cheese dinners
and canned, over-salted soups, not to mention a lifetime of social
drinking, mixed in with an unhealthy addiction to chocolate and
greasy fried chicken. The kids learned early not to get between
Mom and the bucket.

I was starting to think when it came to my health, better to be
safe than sorry. An ounce of prevention was worth a pound of cure.
Catch a falling star and put it in my pocket, save it for a rainy day.

That sort of thinking was reinforced when some of my uncles and
aunts — the ones whose parents had died in a car accident in their
50s — started to face unexpected triple bypass surgeries as they hit
their 60s. Shortly after Mom passed, we got a call that my dad's sister had succumbed to colon cancer. The words "cancer doesn't run
in my family" rang embarrassingly in my ear.

What did I know about anything?

An appointment to see a surgeon for the scope was made via
my usual doctor. For Canadians with Medicare it's cheaper to see
a surgeon than a psychic. It was a tempting idea though. A psychic
could possibly tell me a lot faster what was coming down the pipe,
so to speak.

Sometime in January 2010, I returned to Sandi's office for my
annual Pap smear and breast exam. A "lump with a tail" in the left
breast, discovered through self-examination more than a year ago,
was still causing us concern. Due to the density of my breast tissue,
a possible result of my fond association with large glasses of red
wine, the mammograms and follow-up ultrasounds were not sug-

gestive of any breast cancer patterns. But I was not comfortable with that. My radar was up from Mom's recent passing. I kept pushing. "What *is* it, then?" All I wanted was a simple answer: It's a plugged duct, a lesion, a thickening from an injury . . . a hard elbow shot to the boob that I'd possibly forgotten about?

Sandi referred me to Dr. P, one of three visiting surgeons that rotate scheduling at the Smithers hospital and the one who would be doing my colonoscopy. Dr. P discussed the scoping procedure and then moved on to the left breast lump issue. After doing a physical exam he said, "It doesn't feel anything like a cancerous mass. Whatever it is, I'm very sure it's not cancer."

What can you say to that? It's what we all want to hear. So why wasn't I happy?

"I can take it out if you want."

That widened my eyes. It was the first time I realized there might be a surgery involved here. What? Cut my boob? Whoa, Mr. Scalpel Happy . . . let's just back up a minute here.

It's stupid when you think about it, which is what I'd never done. Stopped and thought all this through. If it was cancerous, there would be repercussions but I never once followed that scenario to the next step.

"I'll have to see," I told him. My skin was sweaty. I would have to consult with Sandi when and if I decided to talk about it. *Surgery? Good grief!*

I got the call from the hospital booking department in February. My colonoscopy was scheduled for May. The calendar seemed to be filling with medical appointments and I was a pre-senior by 15 years. Bette Davis once said, "Old age ain't no place for sissies." Maybe she should have said, "Any age ain't no place for sissies."

Now it was time for my annual mammo. Off to Smithers I went, happy to find a newer mammography machine. This one didn't hurt as much as they lifted my nippled grapefruit onto a plate before closing in on it with another plate. It squished flat like fresh roadkill, only missing the tire marks. Other arm up over my head, get in closer if you can. There, right there. Don't move!

The tech ran into an adjoining room with a view that looked out at the person caught by a boob . . . and took her pictures.

"Cheese," I said to no one. Goosebumps appeared on my naked upper torso. I wondered about all the breasts this woman had looked at . . . big, tiny, floppy, oval, healthy and diseased. Could she tell anything by appearances? Was she looking at mine with a worried expression or was that just her normal face?

She returned and we did it all again on the other side.

Assuming I was finished for another year, I was surprised when the X-ray department called a few days later. I needed to return because there was "something." The radiologist requested an ultrasound, but for the *right* breast. Paste another red doorknob here.

A week later, I lie on the ultrasound examining table telling the technician that she had the wrong side. It was the left breast we were concerned about.

"Really?" She seemed puzzled. "We'll do them both just to be sure. It's standard procedure anyway."

How inept the medical process can be sometimes, I thought. (Smack me with the red doorknob here.)

The results were recorded and sent to a radiologist who would read them and send a detailed report to Sandi.

Another week tumbled away and I was back in Houston at Sandi's female clinic. She had the radiologist's experienced opinion on what he had observed and it was as murky as ever.

"Something shady in the right breast. Suggest another mammo/ultrasound in six months."

I wanted to scream. Frustration soared to an all-time high and my friend could see it.

"I know it's not what you wanted to hear," she told me.

We had been over the option of surgically removing that hard little pea in the left breast. It would mean the end of holding my breath but it was such an invasive decision, especially after the surgeon was so confident it was nothing. And then there was the mix-up with the shadow on the right breast, which to me was totally confusing. The lump was on the left. I put the right breast out of my path of concern.

"There's one other thing we can try. As your breast tissue is extremely dense and there seems to be a reason for further investigation, we can ask for an MRI but that's not something I can refer you for. We have to go through a surgeon again for that."

Dr. P was from Kamloops, so I would have to wait to see him about the MRI the next time he was back in Smithers. I haven't explained it yet, but we live in Houston, a town of 3,500 brave souls living 40 minutes east of the nearest hospital. Smithers, our neighbour with a population of 5,000, hosts the Bulkley Valley District Hospital, an airport, movie theatre and all the major fast food chains. It also has a Blue Fin Sushi Bar, which makes up for anything else our part of the world is lacking. Like designer shoe stores and a drive-thru Starbucks.

Smithers sits beneath the groomed ski slopes of Hudson Bay Mountain. Every time I need a mammo, ultrasound, surgical consult, or some other medical surprise, it would be to Smithers or the even larger centre of Terrace (home of three shoe stores yet still no drive-thru Starbucks) another two and a half hours west of Smithers that I would travel.

It takes a few weeks for Sandi's referral to catch up with Dr. P, but when we meet he is brief. "If that's what you want — and you would have to make your own way down to Vancouver and back — then let's do it."

As far as I'm concerned, my great friend Dr. Sandi Vestvik saved my life that day. At the very least, my right boob owes her its somewhat diminished existence and then some.

The breast MRI was done in the big, wonderful, exciting city of Vancouver, a two-hour flight or 14-hour drive from our area. There is an MRI machine in Terrace and in Prince George, a three and a half hour drive east, but at the time neither were equipped to do breast MRIs.

I was excited to be getting closer to the end of my two-year quest to find out what was in that left breast. Finally some answers. I packed lots of clothes and on May 2nd I kissed my husband good-bye and boarded a plane in Smithers. I tried to relax and look down at the snow-capped mountains as we made our bumpy way up and over the Coast Range. Throughout the rest of the day I travelled by sky train, bus and ferry to North Van and checked myself into a budget hotel for the night, still refusing to acknowledge what might be travelling down the road with me.

3

The Other Boob

After waking and showering in a strange motel room, I dragged my suitcase up and down hills for 50 minutes to get to the hospital. It was sunny but chilly, especially with the perspiration rolling down my back. The exercise felt wonderful and soothing, especially before being seated in another stark waiting room. I found the right department and was given two plain blue hospital gowns (one to conceal my back and one for the front) and slippers before being led to the room where I hoped, finally, to get my answers.

The MRI machine, a massive round donut with a slab table resting horizontally in the middle, seems to occupy most of the room. I sit on the slab while an IV, used for dye injection, is started in my left hand.

"You've done this before," I joke as the nurse expertly slides the needle into a vein, uncaps the port and hooks me up to a bag of saline. It seems as natural as blinking for her.

"My first since I gave up coffee." She grins at my reaction.

I struggle into a prostrate, flying-Superman pose, arms stretched overhead, toes and face down, breasts guided into wide, loose brackets. Headphones are placed on my ears, the voice inside explaining what is about to happen. A small rubber "escape ball" is placed in my left hand.

"It's in case you can't take it," the muffled voice in my ears tells me, "and you need to stop. You squeeze the ball and we will bring you right out, ruining whatever test we are in the middle of." The tech lets the seriousness of what she has said hang in the air between us.

Okay, do not squeeze the ball. That is clear. What isn't clear is what the "it" is. What could be so terrible I would need an escape ball in the first place?

Gears whir and I feel myself travelling backwards, deep into the bowels of the machine. It seems like a giant cigar tube and I am rolled to the very end of it.

PLEASE do not put the lid on while I'm in here!

"The tests will take a total of 45 minutes. The first will be three minutes. Don't move."

My face is supported by a soft padded ring, and a mirror has been placed below so I can almost see a large window with what might be a technician seated behind it. A slight flick of the eyes to the right and I can see a wall clock. I watch the hands go round and round.

Three minutes take so long to pass I wonder if the clock batteries are dying. Or maybe there's been a power outage? Things like that happen. Is anybody still out there? My anxiety rises with the boops, bings and bangs the machine makes around me. It's nerve-racking, a tin can band straight from hell.

Perspiration collects on my forehead. I have been in the tube less than two minutes.

Claustrophobia is a strange sensation. I never felt it during the brain MRI I had in 2002 after the TIAs, possibly because I was laid out on my back. Little mirrors were attached so that I could see very well from inside the long cigar tube. And I could breathe easily. Not so with the breast MRI. You cannot draw a full breath. You are lying directly on your diaphragm, without the pillowy uplift of your breasts. They're in holes, remember? So for the first time since being 13, I was lying flat. I was inside a hot cannon waiting for someone to light the fuse. Where was my helmet? The noises filtering through the headphones were driving me over the edge; I worried I'd been abandoned. I needed to breathe. Just one full breath.

The bopping noises stop for a second. I must be between tests. I squiggle and am rewarded with a deep gulp of air. Finally. Ahhh.

"Don't move!" a voice from the earphones reprimands me.

"But I can't breathe," I whine.

"Twenty minutes to go," I hear back.

I fervently remind myself these tests will answer my most troubling questions. After cancer wrapped its icy fingers around Mom's pancreas, those questions are never far from mind. If this is cancer, I want it dealt with now.

The tests end. The tech congratulates me on my patience and we talk for a minute about how the design of the machine might be enhanced to alleviate this appalling breathing problem. She says they put small, thin pillows above the breast area for one woman who could not stand it. I have since talked to other women who admit they squeezed that ball.

(Magic Mike, my physiotherapist, is amazing at figuring out how to relieve physical discomfort. He suggested raising the hips. During my next MRI, the techs obliged and placed foam wedges beneath my hips which worked perfectly. Extra padding had been added to the gurney as well, dropping the bother level to "slightly inconvenienced.")

I waited while the tech checked to ensure the test results were legible, and then I was free to leave. I questioned her about when I would see the results and was disheartened to hear it would take two weeks. I had been under the impression something might have been done that day.

I returned to the airport, more than a little crushed, with another two-week wait ahead of me. A couple of mini bottles of wine on the two-hour flight home helped my attitude a bit. Hey, I told myself. It had already been two years of suspense. What are two more weeks?

My next fun date with the medical establishment was colonoscopy day. The worst part was a total cleansing of the bowel. This means fasting the day before and drinking a potent little concoction that cleans you out slicker than a brand new rain gutter.

Well, at least I could breathe.

On May 25, 2010, minutes before that scope was performed, I was ushered into the surgeon's office to discuss the results of my MRI, which had just arrived. Dr. P said the mass on the left breast was normal-looking BUT there was something suspicious-looking in the right breast he felt should be pursued.

He then lost me by expounding on options and the next steps we should take and I swear I never heard a thing. I was fuming. What was with these people and the right breast? Did I have to scream it out? It was my left breast, the frigging *LEFT* one, people.

Had I flown all the way to Vancouver and back for nothing?

Dr. P was looking at me with a frown on his face.

What?

" . . . another surgeon will be here in the next few weeks and I'll be turning your case over to him . . ."

What?

"Don't worry; you'll get a phone call from the booking office for an appointment."

"Another surgeon? You're quitting on me? Was it something I said?"

That got a laugh. "No, of course not. I won't be back in the north for a month so I'm giving your file to someone who will be here. He's an excellent doctor. You'll like him. And now . . ." Dr. P pointed toward the door. "I have to prepare for your scoping. I'll talk to you again right before the anesthetist puts you out."

He quickly left the room.

I sat there a minute mulling everything over. Okay, put it out of your head, I told myself firmly. I had more pressing matters going on at the moment. Like where I was going to place all the funny stickers I had bought to cover my ugly white butt, stickers that said "No holding," "No fumbling" and a big one that said "Trust." If you don't know what a colonoscopy is, it's where they snake a camera up through your anus into your large intestine looking for polyps or cancers or any irregularities. I felt sorry for the doctors and nurses having a job that forced them to stand there and look at someone's backside. So, I decided to cover mine with stickers. I had to get the stickers in place before being wheeled into the operating room. I was later told you could hear the surgical team laughing down at the nurses' station.

The scoping went as planned and I got a clean bill of health . . . at that end anyway.

On June 2 I waited in the next surgeon's temporary office in Smithers. From Terrace, he had spent his Wednesday morning performing surgery before hopping in his vehicle, backpack in hand, and driving to Smithers to see more patients.

A bit behind, no pun intended, Dr. Q barreled into the examining room where I sat draped in a hospital gown. I was in my usual grumpy mood, wondering why yet another person had to inspect my breasts.

Wasn't the MRI a be-all and end-all? Didn't we now have all the magical answers? Couldn't someone just tell me what I needed to hear?

Dr. Q introduced himself as he crossed the space between us, his hands already outstretched to reach up behind my neck for the ties at the back of my dressing gown.

My eyes went candy-apple wide.

He stopped abruptly and took a large step backward.

"Did you want a nurse to be present for this exam?" he asked.

And without waiting for my reply he left the room, returning minutes later with the operating room booking nurse.

In my defence, the man could have been the janitor saying he was a doctor. As I said before, what did I know? Well, I didn't know Dr. Q, he didn't know me and all that was soon to change.

Turns out Dr. Q didn't simply want to examine my breasts. He wanted me to bend over and let them hang, cow and udder style. It was humiliating, but he never noticed, too busy looking at them like he was an artist. He was searching for dimpling, a possible sign of breast cancer.

And this is where we experience the least shining moment of my life. Dr. Q suggests I travel to Terrace for yet another ultrasound with the new radiologist, Dr. H. I stoop low, put on my imaginary tiara and play the "Miss Inconvenienced" number. "Go all the way to Terrace?" I ask, as indignantly as possible.

Okay, I admit it was uncalled for but I was so tired of going through the seemingly never-ending hoops, past Sandi and Dr. P and an MRI and then Dr. Q and now to see a Dr. H. When was it all going to end?

In Dr. Q's defence, he is an extremely busy man, a man I came to greatly appreciate and admire but at that moment he was still someone standing between me and what I wanted. And what I wanted was for someone to say, "The end. This disruption in your life is now over. Resume lifestyle immediately. Pass GO. Collect $200. Heck, collect nothing. Just have a great day 'cause you're okay, OK?"

Of course he didn't say any of that. What he said was "What?" with a shocked look on his face, like he couldn't believe what I'd just said to him. He had just driven "all the way" from Terrace to come to see me. Then very quickly, his face changed and he blurted out, "Would you prefer to have a mastectomy?"

Colour that doorknob a flashing RED, RED, RED!

But no, I never heard that clue either. Zing. Right over the fluffy, dyed-blonde hair. (A good colour choice for me at this point, don't you think?) I was stunned. A mastectomy? Whatever for? Where was this man coming from? Mars? Good grief, everyone, let's calm down. You needn't be so rash. I looked over at the nurse to give her a "what's with this guy" smirk but her eyes were now wider than mine. Guess maybe Dr. Q wasn't known to lose his cool. My dad always said I could bring out the worst in even the calmest people (this from a man that has been banned from local yard sales).

The doctor and I stared at one another. I realized this could go one of two ways, and neither of them looked good for me. I mean, really, who goes around annoying someone who might soon be waving a scalpel over their flesh?

And it's not like this wasn't a lesson I had already been taught. I took on a battle-axe nurse in 1985 while in labour with my son. She was determined to shave my pubic area, something that hadn't been done 14 months before with the birth of my daughter. It was the same doctor so go figure! The nurse insisted the doctor had ordered it. I called her bluff. She came at me with the razor anyways, and the result was a hack job that left me walking funny for a week.

Possibly that story helped cool me off because I backed down, removed the tiara and agreed to go to Terrace for a biopsy of the stupid shadow on my right breast.

But while I'm there, will someone please get to the bottom of that left breast issue? I didn't care that the MRI said it looked fine. It was still a round hard pea and I was positive it had to be something. Who cared about the right breast? I didn't feel a thing in that one.

It was a sunny drive to Terrace. We made good time and arrived ahead of schedule. I checked in at hospital admitting and walked down the hall to the ultrasound area where I met a wonderful technician I will call Angela. That's not her name but it suits her quite well.

Once settled into a pastel yellow hospital gown — much cheerier than the blue ones, I was thinking — I got ushered into a tiny closet of a room and was introduced to this new radiologist, Dr. H. We traded small talk and then the doctor and the tech took a look at the mysterious shadow that was causing all the bother.

The ultrasound wand hovered in one spot over my right breast.

"There is something there." Dr. H looked closer at her computer screen, the image moving with the wand. "Yes, that should be biopsied." There was no doubt in her voice. "You will have to make another appointment for that."

I sat upright, one hand holding the drape cloth to my chest. "What?"

Dr. H was reaching for the doorknob when she stopped and looked back at me.

"Really?" I asked. "I just drove three hours to make this appointment and you're saying I have to come back another time? I was told you would be biopsying it today."

The tech and the doctor exchanged surprised glances.

"Who told you this?"

I said nothing, but my top lip quivered. I could feel anger and desperate disappointment overwhelm me.

Another exchange of glances.

"Please," I said. "It's been so long already. I don't think I can stand another waiting sentence."

I looked from one of them to the other.

"My next appointment cancelled," Angela volunteered. "I'm free for the next 20 minutes."

We both looked at Dr. H.

"Okay. Let's do it," she said.

I lay back down on the exam table before they changed their minds.

The larger room used for biopsies was occupied so the closet we were in would have to do. Angela went to get the biopsy "gun."

At least that's what it looked like to me. It had a handle like a gun and a long barrel that slimmed into a rather large, pointed needle. My grandma had used the same size needle to knit socks. It was extremely evil-looking, right out of Frankenstein's laboratory.

EEK.

The ultrasound wand went back across my breast to relocate the exact position of the shadow. Once found, it was marked and a regular needle plunged in an anesthetic to numb the area. The larger biopsy needle was inserted. Dr. H pulled the trigger and we heard a gunshot of sorts. I felt a burn inside my chest. Small but manageable.

I grimaced but said I was okay when asked.

The knitting needle was withdrawn and held over a small pill bottle filled halfway with clear liquid. The captured specimen was dropped into this. It resembled a tiny pollywog, only a white one with bloody red streaks on it.

Dr. H turned toward me with the gun poised again. A second specimen was taken but not before a second dose of anesthetic, just in case. Before the fourth attempt, the gun fell apart. The technician put it back together, saying it had already been in once for repairs. As Dr. H reinserted the needle for the fifth and last time, she asked again how I was doing. Mid-sentence of trying to say, "I'm fine. I hardly feel a thing . . ." I had to clench my teeth. My breath left me while my knees involuntarily snapped into my chest. A ragged edged bite had been ripped from the centre of my life force, from my soul. If I could have, I'm sure I would have screamed.

"The area is very close to the chest wall. I'm sorry about that, but I think we got it," said the doctor.

Angela's eyebrows were slanted in concern. No one wanted to see anyone suffer around here. When I caught my breath, I surprised them both with gratitude and a thank-you for going ahead with the biopsy in the first place. They could have made me come back and I wasn't about to forget that over a painful jab. It would pass and indeed it did within minutes. I'd had two children, I reminded myself. This was nothing.

It usually took two weeks to get results from a needle biopsy but fate, and Angela, had been kind. Two days after the trip to Terrace we were travelling to Invermere in southern B.C. where my brother Danny lived. Kim was flying in from Ottawa and, together with our families, we were going to scatter Mom's ashes from the top of a mountain.

It was a 14-hour drive so we stopped in Kamloops to visit overnight with some great friends, Barb and Craig. Sandi knew I would be away for a week so I was surprised to see a call from her on my cell phone. Maybe she thought I was still at home and wanted to go for a jog?

I told Barb I had to make a call as she poured me a large glass of Merlot. I stepped out onto her patio and rang Sandi's number. She picked up almost immediately.

Sandi didn't beat around any bush. Pun intended. She told it like it was, apologizing for telling me this over the phone. It's not something she would normally do, but I needed to hear this and deal with it right away.

"Deb, the results are back from your biopsy. It came back positive for invasive ductular carcinoma (IDC). It appears you have breast cancer. I'm so sorry."

For a split second I was speechless, but I recovered quickly, cracking a few jokes, laughing. My laughter had everyone in the house sure the news was good. Sandi rattled off Dr. Q's cell phone number, saying he wanted to hear from me right away to book surgery. I assured my friend I was okay, thanked her for the call and pressed *End* on the phone. Without taking a breath I dialed the number I had been given.

There was no thought about anything other than doing what I was told. Next step. Surgeon. Cut it out. I'd trusted Sandi with my life for years. If she advised this was what I needed to do, then I was headed that way. We would talk more when I got home.

Dr. Q, the man I performed the shameful Royalty Act for, was on holiday but he took my call. You could hear family chatting easily in the background while he explained that we should have the tumour, a 9 millimetre bombshell no bigger than the nail on my pinkie finger, removed as soon as possible. IDC could spread quickly. Once in the lymph node system it could access the rest of my body. When could I come to Terrace again?

What's a lymph node? I wondered.

We decided on a date to meet, both of us willingly cutting our holidays short. I thanked him with a sincere but very flat voice. I headed back inside.

"Good news?" Barb asked.

"I'm not sure," I said. "Depends on how you look at it." I drained the wine in my glass and held it out for a refill.

The good news was they found it in the first place. Nine whole millimetres. It might not have been found a year earlier. It was what they called a mini tumour. I was "lucky," someone said. Probably someone with a much larger mass. I was lucky because there was a chance Dr. Q could save my breast. He would do what's called a lumpectomy or, in my case, a partial mastectomy. Instead of merely removing the lump, they remove a wide swath around the tumour, trying to get any wisps spreading out from the mass. Think of a fried egg. The cancer is the yolk so they take a large portion of egg white at the same time if your breast is big enough. The only other option was a full mastectomy.

Holy crap. Was this really happening?

It took a while to sink in though I'm still not sure it has, or that it ever will, completely. At that moment I swept it under a rug in my head, unsure of what this meant for me. All I knew was that I had a bit of cancer inside of my breast and the surgeon was going to remove it. What was so big about that? I had cancer. It would be gone soon. End of story, right?

I think the biggest realization came when we returned home to Houston and a best friend sent me flowers. What? Was I that sick? Maybe this was going to be worse than I'd imagined? Funny . . . I didn't feel sick. I felt more annoyed than anything.

We all knew how healthy I was. There's the shocker. I had never been in better shape. I ate veggies, fruit and organic meats. I pumped iron, took vitamin supplements. Why was this happening to me? And why couldn't I reach my mother on the phone to tell her about it?

When the "why me" voice subsided I realized this was all because of an insistent non-cancerous growth in my *left* breast which turned out to be an amazing flag. What if I'd never pushed for more answers? What if I'd never gone for that MRI?

Spreading Mom's ashes weighed heavily in light of the breast cancer diagnosis. On the outside I responded appropriately enough. I hugged and joked with our adult children, who had gathered in a rental home in Invermere for the weekend. There was joy in catching up with their daily soap operas, watching them laugh and interact with one another. Having my sister around, my niece and nephew, my brother with his wife . . . everything was together for me. Yet inside I was a cyclone of questions and uncertainty, not sure whether to light a candle and learn to pray or just get very, very drunk. What was going to happen to me? Was I about to follow Mom? Was fate miraculously giving me a chance to say goodbye to everyone gathered? Would it be fair to add my black cloud to Mom's final parade?

No, that would turn the weekend into something about me. My sister's words rang in my ear. "You aren't always the centre of everything." She was right. Mom deserved to have this day for herself.

My determination to keep the news lasted five minutes. One look from my sister, that unspoken "What's the matter now?" as she furrowed her eyes at me, had the beans spilled.

My brother also figured something was up between the looks Kim and I kept exchanging.

They cornered me in the kitchen.

"I didn't want to say anything yet," I hedged.

"Anything about what?" My brother casually picked up a carrot stick to chew on.

"Tell him," Kim said.

"Tell me what?"

"You tell him," I said.

"Tell me what?"

"No, it's your news and you should be the one to tell it." My sister pointed two fingers at my eyes then back at her own eyes. Focus, it said. I hated when someone did that to me, and she knew it.

"Okay, fine, alright, I have breast cancer, satisfied?" I glared at Kim. I couldn't look at Danny yet.

"And she's going to be fine," my sister said, grabbing my shoulders and giving me a playful shake.

My brother's face was grave but his head was nodding agreement. It took a minute before he said, "You're a fighter, Deb. I feel sorry for the cancer. It won't know what hit it."

The moment was interrupted by our kids, aged 13 to 30, but not before we agreed I would wait a week before telling the next generation. That way I could talk to each of them separately, over the phone.

I was a walking wuss of a mother, the epitome of how not to parent. But the choice suited me at the moment. When in doubt, procrastinate. It's a major sign of ADD.

The Saturday was all blue skies and sunshine as we climbed to a majestic clearing to liberate Mom's powdery remains. A paraglider attached the container to his belt and then radioed us from overhead to say the ashes were being released. We cheered as she drifted on the wind.

On Sunday we returned to our separate lives, promising we would face my diagnosis together. It was a fretful goodbye with ultra bear hugs. That big-C word has a way of scaring the living daylights out of everyone. I was beginning to get the picture. This was serious.

Breaking news of this magnitude to your children is never easy. You can't tell how they will react. My daughter Karly took it the worst, which is to be expected. Now an adult living away from home, Karly was by herself when I dropped the stinker. It made me regret my decision not to have told her in person. I would have been there to console her. But no, I had been worried about not being able to put on a brave front, which made me a double coward. Karly kept repeating the word *no*, like I had for Mom. I wished I could reach through the phone and hold her. Damn my scattered brain. I should have thought this through better. All of my own uncertainty was reflected in her voice. I know Karly didn't think of it at the time, but my diagnosis increased her possible risk of breast cancer.

I responded to her concern with "I'm fine, things will be fine" and lie, lie, lie, joke, joke, joke. Karly suggested I start writing and blogging everything so people could keep track of what was happening. It was a wonderful idea I quickly considered.

Lindsay put on a brave face considering she lost her mother to lung cancer in 2000. She wished me strength and positive thinking, promising to research safer skin care alternatives through her health professional job at a drugstore.

My son and stepson are men. "Keep us posted. Cheer up. You'll get through this." That's what I thought too. This would be over as quick as you could say "a week on the couch." Right?

When, I asked myself, *when have I ever been right?*

It is what it is. You can run, but you can't hide.

Without my really being aware of it, my cancer journey had begun. My name had been given to the Smithers Community Cancer Service, and Nurse Alice phoned to invite me for a chat and to give me some information booklets I might find interesting. I think Alice holds one of the most difficult jobs in cancer care. She's the one that gets the "DPs" — the dazed and panicked people. We stumble to meet her in shock. We have questions no one can answer . . . Why me? What happened? What *will* happen?

Alice was a buoy and I clung to her like a petrified kid in the deep end of the pool for the first time. "Don't let go, don't let go, don't let go!" She made me feel she personally would make sure I went through this journey with all the help and comfort and care that was possible. I left a little less panicked, with a tiny bit of confidence that I would survive. Under my arm was tucked a new plastic folder containing the *Breast Cancer Companion Guide* and calendar and another handy workbook called *Living and Learning*. Small in size, *Living and Learning* is a lighthouse in importance. It explained the "what comes next" with compassion and gentleness and was peppered with quotes from author Carol Shields regarding her own fight with breast cancer. The book encouraged me to keep notes, so I bought myself a purse-sized spiral notebook where I began to record everything. I taped in a page of phone numbers I continually added to as the treatments changed. One side had medical numbers. The flip side had contact info for friends and relatives. Then I started writing down everything that had happened since discovering the left breast lump. I got Sandi to help me fill in the dates of the mammos and ultrasounds. This record came in handy when talking with the oncologist.

I learned I had the right to ask for the reports on any medical tests to keep for my own records, which I did. The notebook also came in handy for remembering the names of people I met on my cancer journey, tips from magazines and even the recipe for a lemon meringue pie martini. Once I finished treatment I flipped back to the recipe and made sure I tried one . . . and just one. My pre-cancer self would probably have had four.

Alice clarified that along with the cancer the surgeon would be removing some sentinel lymph nodes. Dye is injected into the bloodstream and tracked to those nodes closest to the tumour, following the path cancer cells may have taken. Those nodes would then be removed and checked for cancer. When I still looked confused she described a lymph node as one of many small pods in the body that filter bacteria, cancer cells, and other foreign material travelling through our extensive lymphatic system.

If the cancer inside of me were to spread, it would end up in a

lymph node. The number of nodes containing cancer would deter-
mine the type and length of cancer treatment.

I was also told the lymph node surgery would bring major and
permanent changes in my life. I would have to stop carrying heavy
things with the arm on the affected side and be extra cautious about
the risk of injury or cuts, burns or infections. Blood pressure cuffs,
IVs and needles on that side should also be avoided. The worry was
lymphedema. That's where your arm swells up and, if not caught in
time, it could be permanent.

When you lose sensation in an area due to surgery, it's difficult to
tell how hard you are pressing with a razor blade and you risk piercing the skin. As I shave my underarms, it was suggested I buy an
electric razor. And it is best to buy your own. Then you don't have
to be like me and buy another one when you ruin your husband's.

An interesting section of the *Living and Learning* book was titled
"Understanding Breast Cancer." It expanded on breast cancer risk
factors. Based on research from 1,000 women, your risk was lower
if you were 14 years of age or older when your menses started, you
were younger than 20 for your first full-term pregnancy, you were
thin (does it count if you have to fight to keep it that way?), you
breastfed for six months or more, you never used hormonal contra-
ceptives or hormone replacement therapy, you came from a "low-
socio-economic status" (what . . . drinking the more expensive wine
was worse for you?), you lived in a rural community (bingo!) and
you came from Asian ethnicity.

Okay, I was 13 on the menstrual question, 24 for the first child, try
five months for the breast feeding and who knew what was in that
spermicidal jelly? I received one small check mark for living rurally.
They must be assuming we ate farm-fresh eggs, organic meats and
vegetables. I got another small check mark for the organic meats.
But that didn't mean all the meat I ate had been hunted. My husband
brought home wild grouse, fish, moose and deer but when chicken

or ribs went on sale, I stocked up on the hothouse-born, overfed and possibly pesticide- and fertilizer-laced meats, just like everyone else.

The highest risk factors were being over 50 (bingo), born in North America or Northern Europe (bingo), having two immediate relatives with breast cancer, having a previous cancer or being a person with the BRCA1 or BRCA2 genes (BReast CAncer susceptibility genes 1 and 2).

Moderate risk included having dense breast tissue (another bingo), and if you've ever had a high dose of radiation to your chest (bingo: two CT scans after the strokes).

Late menopause confers higher risk than earlier. Being 12 or younger at menarche is the number one moderate risk factor and being slim trumps being overweight in the low risk category.

Oh my head. I felt like a gopher running here, running there.

What had happened to me? Who was responsible? My gene pool? My waiting to have children until I was 24? My urban, high-socio glass of red wine? That chicken and Italian sausage casserole we loved once a week? Who can tell? You could win the lucky life lottery or the lousy life lottery. All we really know is that everyone's got tickets.

If that's not enough to depress you . . .

So what do I do when I'm depressed? I do something that makes me feel good. Listening to inspirational music definitely helps. From Pink's "Raise Your Glass" to Gloria Gaynor's version of "I Will Survive" or my favourite "Ordinary Day" by Great Big Sea (the lyrics are in Appendix F), I jump to the beat around the living room and things get better instantly.

If that fails, I phone a friend.

Third choice comes in a wrapper.

4

The Inevitable Fall

On August 9, 2010, my husband and I booked into a Terrace hotel. We were to see Dr. Q first at the hospital for a pre-surgical examination. He asked to see us in the emergency room where he was working on call.

I was seated on a gurney, stripped to my waist beneath a hospital gown when the good doctor appeared, his son following close behind. His son is also a doctor, training to be a surgeon, and was in Terrace on holidays. He came to job shadow. I didn't mind getting two experienced doctors for the price of one.

During the examination, I asked Dr. Q once more about my left breast, the one I had been concerned about since the very beginning. He decided to aspirate it on the spot, using a fine needle to draw out some cells from the lump. His son asked me a few questions. "Do you smoke? Do you drink?" And I gave my usual answers . . . no and moderately.

It wasn't until I got home that I started to think about those two questions again. I had smoked. Smoked for 21 years and had quit 13 years ago. A pack a day of nicotine and carcinogens should have given me lung cancer ages ago. But I had made it through . . . hadn't I?

A nameless girlfriend who found out I had breast cancer quipped, "Oh right, you used to smoke. I'm safe," she said. "I never smoked." The "you did this to yourself" was never said but I felt it hanging in the air.

Shame on me. What had I done to myself in those years?

As for drinking, the "moderately" added up to around 20 to 30 drinks a week. I admit it was hard to sit myself down and count that out. I had to be brutally honest, counting the liqueurs in the two blueberry teas we traditionally had in the ski cabin every Wednesday before we hit the lounge. Add another three large glasses of wine before sashaying back to the cabin for another glass of wine with dinner. On Thursday the party started at 4 p.m. in the lounge. Free appys and door prizes sponsored by local businesses. Add three drinks there, three more in the evening. That's six. We enjoyed drinks on the deck with our BBQ lunch, après-ski drinks before drinks with our company over and after dinner.

How many calories was that? No wonder I had to work so hard to keep the weight down. I busted my butt six days a week to keep it covered in the same-sized jeans month after month. In hindsight (pun intended) all I had to do was cut down on that sugar and alcohol.

Life had been one big party after another. They say "everything in moderation." Was all that drinking considered moderate? I started to think not. I had been the personification of (attempted) suicide by grapes!

Most cancer books try to talk you out of blaming yourself. They're quick to say it can never be proven it was the alcohol or the progesterone pills, the toxins in your hair products, the stress or the charbroiled steak fat that caused the cancer. So maybe we don't know what spawned that first cancerous cell but we do know what helps it multiply. You can minimize the chance of a recurrence with this knowledge. You can also warn others.

I think a healthy compromise would be in order. Don't try to sort out the exact cause because most likely it was a combination of things that started the cancer. Instead, think about your past lifestyle and omit or re-examine what you think needs to be changed. Anything in excess is bad for you. Eat Oreos and Cheetos, but only as an occasional treat. Everyone has room for ditching a few of their tickets in the cancer lottery.

Your best chance of avoiding cancer and surviving cancer treatments is to lose the booze. The way I understand it, your liver must deal with alcohol before it can deal with anything else. Chemo, radiation, cancer cells, excess hormones from alcohol or body fluctuations due to premenopause stand by and, while doing so, can create havoc. All that extra estrogen from the alcohol and my being perimenopausal (a stage right before menopause) fed my cancer.

The recommended alcoholic consumption for women is no more than one-half to one drink a day (based on 5 ounce glasses of wine or one of any spirit). Once over that, any positive effect alcohol has on your system becomes detrimental. Most men, I'm jealous to say, can handle two a day.

That afternoon I met with Dr. Q at his downtown Terrace office. Sandi and I had discussed my options. This growth had to be dealt with quickly and the best route for me would be surgery. I had a page of questions ready for Dr. Q. Serious stuff, like . . . how many nights in hospital? Could I prearrange no-fat meals? Were there private rooms? How big would the scars be? Would I still be able to wear a bikini?

He answered them with ease. He had travelled down this road many times before. I paused before signing the consent form. Dr. Q noticed I had one question unticked on my list.

His eyebrows rose. "Any more questions?"

I fidgeted.

"What?" he asked. "What did you want to know?" A slight smile tugged at his lip.

Was he daring me?

Warmth flooded into my cheeks, my brain yelled, *No, don't ask* THAT, but I opened my mouth anyway. "The hospital bathrooms, do they have hair dryers?"

I never expected him to laugh at me. I mean really, the question wasn't that preposterous. But the man had to hold his belly, he was laughing so hard. It took a Mexican minute for him to compose himself. "You won't need to wash your hair," he told me, his voice deadpan while his lips remained curled up in a smile. His eyes twinkled with mirth.

Well, I thought in a huff, he may know a lot about surgery, but really, what would this man know about a woman's hair?

Yes, I know, I never ever learn.

At 6:20 the next morning, without usual adornment of makeup or jewellery, I walked through the emergency area of the Terrace hospital. It looked spooky and quiet in the early morning light. Not the usual shuffle of bent, pained-looking people wandering the halls.

Upstairs in the nuclear medicine department I slipped into a hospital gown. All four quadrants of my right breast were injected with blue dye. It's called technetium, a radioactive tracer that gets absorbed into the lymphatic drainage system. It shows the nodes most likely to be concealing cancer cells that may have migrated from the tumour. The tumour, an area around the tumour called the margin and the sentinel nodes are then surgically removed. The excised nodes are frozen, sectioned and examined by a pathologist. As my tumour was so small, chances were good the nodes were clean. Or so I'd read.

In the surgical department I was given an ID bracelet, weighed (149 pounds) and asked about false teeth (they made me prove I didn't have any and I made a big show of opening wide to stick my tongue out at the world) and any prior illnesses or diseases. "Just put down prone to severe chocolate withdrawal symptoms," I said.

Then it was back to nuclear medicine for X-rays showing the path taken by the blue dye and which nodes had to be removed. I carried the images back to the surgery holding area, which gave me a chance to look at them. I was surprised so many were lit up, counting at least five.

Next stop . . . the ultrasound department to have a wire inserted into my breast. The tumour was lying very close to the chest wall, deep inside the breast. A guide wire would make it easier to locate and excise it. But oh, oh. It's Dr. H, now thought of as Dr. H-ouch. The thought went through my head, I could turn around and walk out of the place. No one was going to chase after me. This was all voluntary, right? Wouldn't I rather be sipping a latte at Starbucks? Wouldn't I rather be doing other anything than facing this twisted music?

But I didn't go. I stayed and faced Dr. H-ouch. I explained this was her chance to atone for that painful biopsy she performed weeks ago. She simply smiled at that. There would be no promises. This was a world of "Do whatever is necessary to get the patient through it and out the other end alive." You hope they keep you comfortable while it happens but that's all it is. A hope.

With my permission, a student was allowed to attend. A young girl with long, wavy brown hair stepped into the room, moving back into the shadows but not before nodding a sympathetic smile at me. She stood far enough away that she wasn't hanging over us but was still able to get the gist of what was going on.

It took three injections of anesthetic to get my breast numb enough for Dr. H to proceed and, because my breast tissue is so dense, Dr. H-ouch was finding it difficult to get the long, thin wire inserted. After three attempts, she had the technician, Angela, hold the breast immobile with two hands while she again attempted to drive the wire to the tumour site. With alligator tears rolling, toes clenched and curled, and all breathing stopped, I tried to visualize a beach, a free, all-you-can-eat seafood buffet somewhere, a day at the park with my children. It wasn't working.

The student was told to leave the room. This was getting ugly.

"I suppose failure is not an option," grumbled Dr. H-ouch under her breath. Nope . . . not with surgery pending within the hour. Again and again she tried until I felt a searing pain pierce something deep inside of me. It felt like I had been skewered. Swear words were too trivial and would not help. But the wire was now in place. It stuck out from my breast like a rogue antenna. The immediate area was on fire and I was terrified that I, or someone else, would accidentally hit it. My gown was pulled back on, carefully, and I was at last ready for surgery.

I was told I could walk down the hall to the operating area. Dr. H left the room while Angela stayed behind to clean up. Still barely able to breathe properly, I asked Angela to please leave for a minute. I needed a few seconds alone to pull myself together. But as soon as the door closed behind Angela, my world imploded. Everything I had kept pent up for the past months came unleashed. A waterfall of disbelief and misery splashed down my cheeks. My thoughts swirled with pain, anger and grief. I cried with remorse and sympathy for myself, for anyone having to endure this. Had my mother been in this much pain? That thought added to my agony. What was ahead of me? More of this torture? Was I going to be able to handle this? It all came out in torrents.

Even with my fist shoved deep into my mouth, I imagine the entire ward heard the racking sobs. Angela quietly returned to the room. We both knew the pity party had to end. I was embarrassed. I was made of better stuff than that. The look on Angela's face said something different. What I saw there was a consoling smile, a look that said other women had felt this misery, which was a normal re-action to what I was going through, and it wished me well.

I managed to rein in once more. Stoicism returned to my face even if my lips still quivered and a few tears leaked. Angela got me into a wheelchair and wrapped me in comforting hot blankets for which I will be forever grateful. She then personally rolled me down the hallway toward surgery with the receptionist calling after her that the next appointment had arrived. Angela didn't acknowledge her and continued to steer me out of the ward and down the hall toward the operating room. Halfway there we met two nurses who had come looking for me. I bade Angela a weepy farewell, saying I would be okay in a minute. But my single minutes were dragging into double digits. The nurses helped me into a hospital bed, wrapped me in another warm blanket and left me in the quiet hallway of the pre-surgical area, giving me a needed moment to settle down. Dr. Q wandered past at one point and without saying a word reached out and squeezed my big toe as he continued down the hall. Word spread fast. Such a small gesture, but it was very reassuring.

Once inside the surgical area, I was questioned again by nurses and a grumpy anesthetist who admitted he had been on call and was up part of the night. He wondered about the mini strokes in 2002.

"They now figure they were a result of my taking Ritalin for my ADD."

"And who diagnosed this ADD?" he demanded.

I thought back but drew a blank.

"I don't remember," I told him. "I have ADD, remember?"

A nurse standing by my elbow tried to stifle a laugh.

It's the last thing I remember. I was out faster than you can say "no sense of humour."

They told me later I came out of the anesthesia in the midst of a conversation with my mother. We were arguing about the Ritalin prescription. Mom was against it. I never knew that before.

Where had I been while I was gone?

I was rolled down a hallway and into an unoccupied four-bed

ward. I was grateful for the privacy as my pain medication wasn't working and it took the staff a while to come up with an effective combination.

Barry, my white knight, appeared with a chai tea latte. He didn't say much, which I appreciated. What was there to say? His eyebrows were furrowed but he stood off to the side, watching me make a fuss over the treat he brought.

My first meal arrived, and I realized I was starving. It was well after lunchtime. What a long ordeal the day had been. I inhaled the soup, salad and sherbet and washed it down with the sweet tea. My throat was raw from the breathing tube inserted during surgery. My left arm was hooked up to an IV bag and my right arm was too sore to move very far. That was from the lymph node removal. I was relieved to find the long wire was no longer sticking out of my breast.

I couldn't see any incisions as everything was neatly covered with small, white gauze strips beneath clear, wide surgical tape. I reached up and felt for my breasts. They were both still there. I heaved a huge sigh of relief and heard an echo from my husband. Barry knew how important it was for me to hang on to that flesh. Looking back, it was much like clinging to a teenaged possession. "Hey, it took me years of grief before I got these. No one is taking them away!"

An alternate choice might have been to have a mastectomy, rather than a lumpectomy, and breast reconstruction immediately after. Then no more worries about breast cancer in the affected breast. But that's hindsight for me and a consideration for the next patient reading this.

Reconstruction is a popular choice and can be done at the same time as a partial or full breast mastectomy (removal). It practically eliminates the risk of future cancer and gets you closer to your former self versus waiting for the mastectomy to heal and then proceeding. Reconstruction is also much easier if it is done prior to any radiation, which makes tissue less pliable.

Not a lot of sleep was had that night between beeping sounds and crying from the nursery across the hall. By morning, I was anxious to go home. There was nothing more to do but wait for the pathology report on the excised tissue, which could take weeks. So get me out of here. Please. And no, I did *not* want a shower or a hair dryer. No one even suggested it.

I was dressed within minutes and headed for the door. I got stopped by the nurse.

"Where do you think you're going?"

"I'm making a run for it," I told her with a wry smile.

Her smile matched my own. "And you didn't think I would catch up to you with that hunched-over, post-surgery shuffle happening? You get your butt back in that bed and I'll find Dr. Q to get some release papers signed."

I remained standing, stoned and not able to process anything quickly.

"In bed, now, please. And where, by the way, were you going without Barry?"

Oh, right, I thought. *Wasn't he living in the parking lot?*

"Good point, I'll just wait in my bed."

Before I finished the statement, my husband walked in with hot tea lattes in either hand. Barry had trouble saying how much he cared but he certainly knew how to show it.

It was a groggy ride back to Houston and I was sore under my right arm where the nodes had been removed. The nerves burned, especially when my arm touched the incision line. When we got home I set up camp on the living room sofa, wrapped to my chin in my fave faux fur blanket. The angle of the sofa's back was perfect for keeping the surgical-side elbow up and away from my body. A pre-rented stack of DVDs would keep me distracted.

Except for forcing a daily walk down our half-mile-long driveway, I lived on that couch for seven days and seven nights. When I stood, I held my sore right breast with my left hand and positioned my right hand on my hip to keep it away from the incision beneath my armpit. People called, friends popped by. I sat up but I never strayed far from the couch. It was my world. My rock.

My husband let me be whatever it was I needed to be for the moment. He made our meals unless I felt up to rooting around in the kitchen. He appeared happy to be able to help with something besides driving me to and from appointments.

I realized, maybe for the first time, what a real "man" Barry was. Textbook Mars, right down to the cave dwelling, left-brained boy who tried to communicate with the alien from Venus lying on his couch. Barry wanted to do or say something that would fix me, but knowing how we operated together he decided his best plan might be to stay mute in the background.

He was smart beyond his years. I was thankful for the space, knowing Barry was never more than a loud moan away. Finding it was only from discomfort often brought a look of dismay, but he quickly tried to hide it. Still, he ran in every time, just in case.

"Can you tell me now how you felt?" I asked recently.

Barry rubbed at his lips, a nervous habit to gain time. "Like how do you mean?"

"How did you handle the fact that your wife had cancer and was having to go through some pretty harsh treatment?"

"Didn't you notice I never used the snow blower all that winter? I cleared the driveway by hand so you wouldn't see me falling apart."

I was shocked to hear it. Looking back, I realize Barry should have called the Canadian Cancer Society (CCS) helpline for the support I couldn't give. He could have talked to someone who had been through the experience.

Fast forward another week to my first post-surgical inspection with Dr. Q, this time in Smithers, our mutual halfway ground. No regal act this time. No La-La-Land Hair-Dryer Girl.

"Seems to be repairing nicely," Dr. Q said, inspecting the half-moon circle around my nipple and the bright pink scar beneath my armpit. He sniffed the air. No foul odours came from the incisions; nothing was green or off-looking. My arm was not swollen. I could still crack a joke.

"I think you did a pretty good job," I tell him, "for someone in training."

His face fell an inch and his forehead wrinkled.

"Training to work with prima donnas," I added.

"Oh, trust me," he said, "you were neither the first nor the worst."

"Finally," I replied. "So, what's next?"

"We won't know anything until the pathology report returns. Until then, keep up the good work with the daily walks. It's important to keep moving, even when you don't feel like it."

Five days later yet *another* surgeon I had never met, Dr. F, entered the small interview room at the Smithers hospital. He was the only surgeon available that week and would be delivering the pathology news to Barry and me.

It was a good thing he was a stranger. It was easier to dislike an outsider who shredded our hopes the way this one did. The lump had been successfully removed but with only a 500 micron margin on one side. In layman's terms, not enough egg white around the yolk had been taken out. That was a cause for concern. But the real bomb was that a tiny bit of cancer, two millimetres worth, was found in one of the seven excised lymph nodes. The cancer had metastasized from the breast to another part of my body. It had been caught trying to escape!

That was the *really* bad news.

If it was there, had it managed to get beyond the node?

Dr. F continued matter-of-factly, saying this could mean more surgery, more breast and lymph node removal, possibly chemotherapy, probably radiation. The punches came hard and fast. I watched his lips moving, but I wasn't making a lot of sense out of anything. Did he just say what I thought he said? What was he saying now?

"Any more questions?"

"Uh, yeh. But you know what, I'm going to ask for a copy of that paper in your hand and get Sandi to go over it with me."

"That's fine." Dr. F returned to his desk, asking, "Do you mind if I examine you?" over his shoulder, almost as an afterthought.

"Actually, yes, I do mind. I'm sorry" — I'm so Canadian at times — "but I think my breast has been through enough trauma for the moment, thank you anyways."

This translates as "You'd have to hog-tie me first just to get near me at the moment."

I stood up and left the room, leaving Barry to walk out after me, I'm sure with an apologetic glance toward the doctor. My husband knew what I'd meant.

Queen DebiLyn managed to get out through the hospital's front doors and into the Suburban where I sat in absolute shock.

Once we were on the highway back to Houston, Barry and I did our usual bickering thing.

Me: "More surgery, chemotherapy and radiation! Could this be for real?"

Him: "No, you won't be *having* chemotherapy. The doctor was referring to drugs that curb a recurrence."

"But he said the chemo word, I heard him."

"He didn't actually say you would have to have chemotherapy."

"Well I heard him say something that started with C, and I'm pretty sure it was chemotherapy."

"You're not listening to me, again."

"I'm not arguing with you. I'm just trying to explain why you're wrong. Can we stop for ice cream?"

Barry was thinking of the drug called tamoxifen, an estrogen blocker used to starve any residual breast cancer cells. As it turned out, Dr. F was thinking chemo. Score one for me. For once, I wished I'd been wrong.

Anyway, at that point I was unsure of what anything meant. I spent the next few hours making up cute scenarios, choosing to forget all about any C-words . . . because, as my husband said, I had probably heard wrong. Why would they bring out the heavy stuff like chemotherapy when we were talking about micro-sized cooties? Just a wee bit of cancer in a node probably meant radiation of that area. Right? Maybe they would take more out, right? Or maybe I could skip another surgery and just radiate everything because it was such a wee bit, a small tumour and I was so lucky. Who said I was lucky?

None of this should have been happening anyway.

I could handle having a little bit of cancer. If I had to. I guessed.

Surface Girl came forward again. Let's not get too deep into this situation. We'll just skim the top, float on the river of cancer. No putting our head under water. No sinking towards the truth.

Then I met with Sandi in her office to go over the results. Friend or not, there was no sugar-coating any of it. She got right to the point, looking me straight in the eyes to make sure I was paying attention. Possible full mastectomy of that breast.

My eyebrows shot up to my hairline.

"The surgeon will probably recommend going for that clear margin. The oncologist in Kelowna will look at everything and make her recommendations."

Another piercing gaze into my eyes as she delivered the second part of the news. "And chemo. You will most likely be having chemotherapy. Once they find cancer in a lymph node, it's usually advised."

Tears started to run in rivulets down my cheeks although I wasn't sobbing. I grabbed a Kleenex and dabbed at the water but my voice was steady. I was hyper-focused on every word Sandi said.

"But it was only a *micro* metastasis . . ." was the best argument I could come up with. "Just a *little* bit of cancer . . ."

I had to admit that my reasoning sounded ridiculous, even to me. And really, how could I sit there and dispute a best friend's experienced prognosis?

But I did. I tried to convince Sandi that I was going to be okay, that I would be able to avoid the horror of adjuvant cancer therapy. I wasn't ready to face the thought of any of it, and so it just wouldn't happen. In other words, I was in complete denial, prepared to barter with the devil . . . whatever it took to be spared. Spared *what*, I had no idea. All I knew about chemotherapy was from movies where bald people with dark-ringed eyes and kerchiefs on their heads usually died.

I left Sandi's office fully mopped up, smiling and telling my friend I would see her on the weekend for a jog. I would have to hold the breast firmly with my arm or hand as I ran but I could still run, I assured her.

It wasn't until I got to my vehicle that the reality of what had been said crept up over my shoulder and bit me. Hard. I was probably going to have chemotherapy. It was the scariest thought, right up there with seeing a ghost when I was all alone in a strange place.

And maybe a full mastectomy, I told myself. I might permanently lose a part of my body. One of my breasts. My hand absent-mindedly flew up to touch it.

Chemo. OMG. Chemotherapy. Chemotherapy. I glommed onto the word as I tried to wrap my head around it. Sandi wouldn't have mentioned it if she hadn't figured it might be a possibility. I started my vehicle, trying not to think about anything. Just keep moving. But that didn't work for very long.

Thankfully I have another best friend up the road from the clinic. Instinctively I headed her way. It was a good move. I managed to pull in and turn off the truck before succumbing to great racking sobs. My body started trembling, shaking harder and harder with every sob. I rocked back and forth like I was in excruciating pain and I was, although it was entirely mental, mostly from the fear of it all. Sharon came out of her house and wrapped her arms around me for the longest time before I could get out of the vehicle and stand on my own feet.

Sharon is the embodiment of the anonymous saying, "Friends

are quiet angels who sit on our shoulders and lift our wings when we forget how to fly."

I think I reacted so intensely because I had absolutely no idea what chemo involved. I had purposely skipped over the section on chemotherapy in my stack of breast cancer books. That wouldn't be applying to me. I was determined to remain a *partial* cancer victim; I couldn't let this consume me. I wanted it to be more like a real bad hair day . . . get it cut and get on with life.

But cancer doesn't always work that way. And it sure didn't care what I wished for. So, once again my life went into a holding pattern as I waited to hear from the oncologist. My future was in her hands.

I should explain that we were given a choice of oncologists. The B.C. Cancer Agency (BCAA) has cancer clinics in Kelowna, Surrey, Vancouver, Victoria and, at the time of writing, a fifth one was opening in Prince George. These clinics offer full services with medical and radiation oncologists, nurses, and technicians. Once you decide where you want to go, your information is forwarded to an oncologist at that site. This person guides your care through every part of the journey once a diagnosis has been made. In short, your oncologist is your *new* best friend.

Chemotherapy can now be administered in most hospitals, including Smithers, Terrace and Prince George, but radiation treatments must be given at one of the five major centres. If we had to do any travelling for examinations, or radiation, we'd go to Kelowna. Lindsay and my Uncle Ross live there and the BCAA clinic — the Cancer Centre of the Southern Interior — is just 10 blocks from my uncle's home.

That's how we ended up with the wonderful and very pregnant oncologist, Dr. KJ.

5

Round Two and Still Swinging

As we live a 12-hour drive from Kelowna, Dr. KJ relied upon the assessments and tests conducted by Sandi and Dr. Q. I didn't get to meet my oncologist face-to-face until six months after my initial diagnosis. It felt very strange having someone you'd never met hand down orders that affected your existence. At least with a judge you got to face him. So it was more like what I imagined God to be. You didn't get to meet him, but he could make your life hell if he wanted to . . . in your best interests, of course.

It was September 1st when Sandi broke the news that a second surgery had been requested. The oncologist had asked the surgeon to go back in and get the margin around that fried egg. And while he was at it, he might as well remove more lymph nodes in the chain and see if any of them had been infiltrated. That meant reopening the scars that were only now starting to feel marginally better. Another two to three weeks of life on the couch.

The surgeon's secretary phoned and confirmed with me. We booked a date. Same story, same procedure . . . except this time a drain would be attached to my side to remove the fluid from my over-pillaged lymphatic system. The good news? The breast could still be saved, although it would soon be missing an estimated 50 percent of content.

"Unless the breast collapses," the surgeon added.

This did happen to a friend of mine. She also required a second surgery to widen the margin. Weeks after the procedure her breast deflated, which prompted her to initiate an investigation into breast reconstruction. As for me, it seemed inane to base a decision on whether or not something might collapse. We would deal with that if it happened.

I say we but, as usual, I never consulted with Barry, merely made up my mind and booked the surgery date. Lucky for me, Barry was committed to seeing me through all this without having to add his opinion. He agreed it was my choice. I figured we would need to have another talk when I was out the other side, to see if he still wanted to be tied to this cut-up, cancerous anchor. I know we said "in sickness and in health," but I would never have held him to it. Especially if it ever got worse. The thought depressed me. I realized just how much I loved the guy. Did it really matter about Johnny Horton or the chunky potato salad? Not in a million years.

My "deflated" girlfriend, compliments of our Canadian medical system, will end up with a matching pair of breasts. Once healed, an expander can be surgically inserted beneath the damaged breast area. It contains a fillable bag that is injected with silicone over a period of time. This lets the radiated skin slowly stretch to accommodate a silicone implant that will eventually replace the expander. And yes, they are back to silicone implants, assuring me they are safer than ever before. I think they automatically come with share options in a bridge they're proposing to build across Niagara Falls.

As our surgeon pointed out, if a threat of cancer recurrence was high, both breasts could be removed to eliminate future worry. A new set of breasts would be constructed using the silicone implants or fat from the body. (I had enough to build two sets, I assured him.)

It was an option to consider. It would be nice to end this ordeal with a pair of perky boobs, especially ones that reduced my "waste." Yet who wanted any more surgery in their future?

I was finding it hard to believe I had to go beneath the scalpel again for the cancer, never mind the repair work. I was finally healing, back to jogging twice a week and laps at the pool for 30 minutes. I didn't move fast, but I stuck with the exercise in fear of facing an insurmountable return to my usual routine. If the task was too overwhelming, I might not have the staying power to get back to some semblance of the old Deb.

August 9, 2010, was a spectacular, sunny autumn day. The leaves in the north change early and the trees had turned impossible yellows and oranges. We cruised by, going under the posted 100 kilometres per hour.

"Funny how we speed for you but crawl when it's me that's in a rush," I needled.

Barry kept his eyes on the road.

"I didn't see you sitting in the Suburban ready and waiting."

"I *was* waiting for you," I huffed. "What were you doing?"

"I was making sure we had all your medical records and your suitcase for your surgery tomorrow. What were you doing?"

"Uhhh," I sighed, "I was Googling hikes in Terrace we could do before I have to sign the surgery consent forms at 3 p.m. This is my point. If we don't go faster, I'm not going to have time to hike anywhere before landing back on our couch for another few weeks."

I was leaning over, directing my voice right to Barry's right ear. "Don't you realize how important this is to me?"

A hot flash swept over me and I scrambled to remove clothes and up the air conditioning.

Barry reached out to close his air vents that began blasting everything but snow. "You don't have to get four hours in. A shorter hike will still do the trick."

I fanned myself while pulling at my neckline. "No it won't. I need as much time as I can get to savor the climb, the view, my heart thudding in my chest, the butt burn. I can't return to that couch at home without feeling how alive I can be first. Please!"

The driver side window rolled down five inches, presumably to let some warm summer air in. "You'll feel all that. Stop worrying."

The Suburban signal light went on. We were turning off into a gas station.

"You've got to be kidding me! We have to get gas? Why didn't we leave half an hour ago?"

"Would you have been ready?" he asked, knowing full well the answer.

My arms crossed over my chest. It was a quiet journey to Terrace as I stewed about the smirk on my husband's face. We arrived at the parking lot halfway up Terrace's Sleeping Beauty climb. I burst from the vehicle, pack over my shoulder, and began a march that didn't slow for over an hour. I hiked upward until the guilt over being late for my pre-surgical appointment got the best of me.

"We're so close to the top," I said, bending over, wiping my sweaty forehead with a rag, "but I think I should head down."

"You're going to be late no matter what you do," Barry said, handing me his water bottle.

Call it my mother's work or simple fate, but getting to the surgeon's office an hour late was a good thing. While in his waiting room I looked up from my game player to notice a scrumptious, light-green, leather purse bounce past. It stopped for a minute near the receptionist's desk before turning and parading straight for me.

A voice attached to the purse said, "Deb, what are you doing here?"

I didn't need to look to know it was my friend Jen. "Oh! Hi! Great purse," I told her, with a grin. She was there to see about a lumpectomy which got scheduled for the following week. She would need the dye and the wire and her lump was also a mere 9 millimetres. Wasn't she lucky? she asked. I had to hold my tongue and wished it to be so for her. I meant that with all of my heart. But what fun to run into a friend going through the same challenges. Now I would have someone to compare notes with. Up to now, everything I learned came from doctors, books or the Internet.

The receptionist interrupted our chipmunk chatter and showed me to Dr. Q's office. We got the surgical consent forms signed and went over the biopsy results of the left breast lump; still no answers other than it was not cancerous. Tired of worrying, I asked him to remove it while I was under the anesthetic. Why take chances that it could turn into something one day?

I arrived early the next morning with a basket full of home-baked cookies for the hospital's surgical staff. My logic was to put everyone, especially the anesthetist, in a good mood while I was back under the knife. The second surgery required no invasive, painful wire or nuclear medicine. A different, perkier anesthetist was at my side and before I knew it I was in my hospital room with my own morphine pump, which I used immediately.

With the pain under control, I was fed a liquid dinner. Friends showed up with a chai tea latte, a chocolate sundae, flowers and fresh fruit. Perfect. A sleeping pill put me down for the night even though, yes, more crying babies.

Looking at the drain jutting out of my side made me queasy. There was a clear ball on the end that collected fluid and blood clots which I had to empty down the toilet. There was surgical tape on both breasts holding the skin tightly together. My right nipple looked oddly disfigured, pointing off to the right like a headlight that needed serious adjustment.

At 10 days post-op I was still flat on the couch with eight rented movies stacked beside me. Touching anywhere on the upper right side of my torso hurt. The drain bulb hung disgustingly down my side. Still determined to get back to "me" as quickly as possible, I forced myself off the couch for a daily walk. I attempted chores with rests in between. I had to do something to erase the sympathy bingeing. Like a Kit Kat or an Aero bar, my butt was developing portion-dividing lines.

An even bigger problem was my post-surgery waterbed boob. Filled with liquid, it sloshed with every step. Holding onto it made no difference except that I looked like an idiot walking around with a handful of boob. Dr. Q said the fluid was normal. Things would firm up eventually but meanwhile, no jumping. Okay, I got it. Let the pudding set. Get back on the couch. More movies.

Thank goodness I thought to get my long hair whacked off the week before surgery. My friend Caroline owns a hair salon in the shopping centre. After getting over the shock of my news, she became a co-conspirator in the "turn this rain to sunshine" plan. My sister also got involved, e-mailing me pages of fabulous short hairstyles she was considering. We planned to have the same look but resorted to what our stylists figured would be the best. Kim's face is narrower than mine. Kim's everything is narrower than mine.

At first I wasn't eager to cut my hair. I had finally achieved the perfect 'do and hadn't strayed from the same cut or colour for two years. I loved the silky way it framed my face after I gooped, blow-dried, moussed and gelled it, then waxed it into place. Stunning. I had it down to 15 minutes and it stayed in place most of the day. Now that's good product!

Then I stopped and thought about all the chemicals those products contained. Was I feeding lingering cancer cells with toxins absorbed through my scalp? Was brain cancer going to be added to my list of family cancers?

I began reading the labels on everything, not just food packages. I switched to natural shampoos, conditioners and hair dyes without parabens or ammonia, lotions without SLS, SLES, PG or isopropyl alcohol. It made sense to use natural products with simple ingredients whenever possible.

I had forgotten the boost a new hairstyle could give. The mini pixie felt light and flippy, and I could now wash it myself using the one arm.

My sister sent me a one-handed book holder. I read a lot of books and my one arm would tire quickly. Kim also sent an uplifting, cheerful card every week. It made the goal of reaching the post box more rewarding. But better than all that, she sent our family treasure, a soft, cuddly bear named Homer given to our mother when she was on the palliative care unit. Homer remained by Mom's side until she passed. He became a comfort to Kim and me simply for having been there with us. Homer had seen what we'd seen and silently understood. He was a stuffed animal but it didn't matter. We all bonded somehow. Kim asked if she could take Homer to Ottawa with her and I agreed. She needed him more than I did at the time. She buckled him into the front seat of her rental car and talked to him on her long drive home.

A year later with her busy life threatening to consume her whole, Kim realized she wouldn't be able to come to B.C. while I was going through chemo. So she did the next best thing. Homer arrived via parcel post. I was overjoyed to receive him. I told Kim he was only on loan as I felt a bit like I'd stolen my sister's favourite toy.

That's the wonder of having a sister. Kim always got it. She instinctively knew that while going through treatments, I could squeeze Homer's hand in place of hers and somehow it would be enough. Our stoic furry rock would be there for us through cancer once again.

Three weeks after the second surgery I was able to get a shirt up and over my head! There was a slight "Ow" involved, more like a mouse squeak than an actual yelp. The best part was I could now wear everything in my closet again. It was getting pretty monotonous there for a while, having to stick to button and zipper fronts. I had exactly one item that fit that description so I went thrift store shopping for backup. A thrift store is like a box of chocolates. You never know what you're going to get. The best thing is almost anyone can afford a few "new" items while helping others. It's a win-win.

While in town I was approached by various people I knew. They seemed relieved to see that although I was grey, I was still breathing. The encounters upset me. Maybe I wasn't ready to face the general public at this point? My diagnosis wasn't a secret but I couldn't get home fast enough that day. I put it down to embarrassment I hadn't tried harder to straighten my shoulders or paint more colour onto my face. I had been blogging about my cancer journey. People were watching how I dealt with it.

My underarm area was still very numb although I could feel the surface beginning to thaw. I still used the electric razor rather than a blade because, like a frozen lip at the dentist's, I couldn't feel where the skin to shave began or ended in my armpit.

The surgical scars were healing nicely though two still had scabs. I dotted liquid vitamin E across them before covering them with paper tape. The vitamin promoted healing and the tape prevented stretching, which I read was a problem with the weight of the breast constantly pulling at the scar tissue. Once the scar fades from pink to white, it has healed.

6

The Burning Chemo Question

As promised, Lindsay came through with some valuable info on cancer and nutritional issues. No surprise, but I still needed to hear it, be reminded of it . . . that sugar ranked high as a bad guy.

I was still on the sweet street with the non-alcoholic wine, the daily overdose of "cheer up chocolate," the baking I'd done for visitors, for us, and the chai tea lattes. I was going to have to tighten that up. An Internet article entitled "Ten Studies Showing the Link Between Cancer and Sugar" helped.

Based on results from a seven-year study, it said increased blood sugar levels increased the risk for breast cancer. That article, and another one discussing increased insulin secretion resulting from sugar intake, was enough to make me quit . . . for six days a week. There has to be some fun in life, so back to the "everything in moderation" rule. I finally understood that my perception of moderation wasn't moderate. I wasn't even in the right ballpark.

It will be tough because sugar is practically everywhere. It's in your bread, your peanut butter, your soy sauce, crackers and canned corn. It's even in toothpaste and mouthwash.

You have to start reading labels on every product for disguised sweeteners like sucrose, fructose, molasses, dextrose, turbinado, amazake, sorbitol, and high fructose corn syrup. The World Health Organization suggests that no more than 10 percent of your total daily calories should come from added sugar. The American Heart Association recommends that women eat less than six teaspoons of added sugar every day, and that men should not eat more than nine teaspoons of added sugar. That's about 100 and 150 calories for women and men, respectively. Maybe that doesn't sound like much, but if you drop 100 calories every day, you'll lose about 10 pounds in one year.

Still giving in to your sweet tooth? Start using approved sugar substitutes like stevia, agave syrup, natural honey, dates and maple syrup, anything but refined sugar, white or brown.

Four weeks after going under the knife for the second time my arm was working fairly well but I still suffered occasional sharp pains, more like partial stabs or electric shocks, through the right breast. The doctors call that neuropathic pain. To me they're phantom boob bites. Trying to find a comfortable position for sleeping was one giant coin-toss affair. Obviously sleeping on my stomach or on the surgery side was out of the question, but gravity pulled at the pea-surgery side until my breast ached. Lying on my back brought snores loud enough to wake even me up. I considered buying a soundproof flotation tank but Barry might have had a problem with that in our bedroom.

The liquid, squishing sound inside the breast ended. It felt firmer but I still found it uncomfortable to bounce, skip or run, even if clamping it viselike with my hand. The "I need some couch time" excuse was getting harder for my husband to accept, especially since I was back to jogging.

I still needed to use my good arm for the bulk of what I did. I brushed my teeth with my left hand, stirred, ate and waved with it. When at the gym, I avoided the weights with the right arm. It tired quickly and began to hurt. I did the recommended physio exercises that were listed in the booklet "Partial or Full Mastectomy Discharge

Instructions." Reading it reminded me of how I felt when I got my first book on menstruation . . . I would rather stick pins in my eyes than read this, but something told me I had better do it.

For the exercise, and for that reason only, I resumed many of the household chores. I could fold towels again, wash dishes and make a meal. All in the same day. I even washed the floor using my new one-handed mop. Pretty easy and guaranteed to leave the floors 99.9 percent germ-free just using water. No more chemical cleaners for me.

I got dates to "see" the oncologist November 2 and the radiation oncologist November 3. Since both these people were in Kelowna it seemed reasonable to hope we could meet through the video-conferencing facilities at the Smithers hospital. It's like Skyping — I could see and talk to the specialists in Kelowna and vice versa. I say "hope" because some people in the southern part of our province seem to have difficulty understanding there's a problem with driving 24 hours and 2400 kilometres from Houston to Kelowna for a 15-minute appointment.

"So you're saying you can't make it?" one of them asked indignantly.

I realized I would eventually have to go to Kelowna if radiation was to be part of my treatment. But the question on chemotherapy was still unanswered. The thought of chemotherapy still scared the hell out of me and, like any normal child, part of me was looking for a way out. Another part wanted the chemo drugs in faster than yesterday just in case something had managed to escape through that one cancerous lymph node.

Would I really be comfortable taking a pass on such a cancer-fighting weapon? Was I 100 percent certain the surgeon got it all? Was I certain that radiation plus five years of cancer-prevention drugs would be enough?

These days you don't have to lie sleepless and wonder about such questions. You can grab your housecoat and a warm cup of herbal tea and wander down to the computer, asking a search engine what you want to know. The computer doesn't care if it's four in the morning.

I typed in "Can chemo cause death?" and felt my face fall at the response. Pages of words like "Chemo Kills Patients" and "The Truth About Chemotherapy — It Is Dangerous" scrolled before me. What a start.

It's a fact that chemotherapy has killed people. But were these people on the verge of dying anyway? Or had these people taken the chemo in hopes of recovery and died *because* of it? Chemo is used in palliative care to shrink tumour size enough to alleviate physical symptoms. It also helps slow disease progression.

Worse than merely losing your hair, chemo can weaken your immune system, making you susceptible to whatever bugs you come into contact with . . . like more cooties, some of them worse than cancer. Was I damned if I did and damned if I didn't?

Mom turned it all down, definitely not wanting to prolong the agony. She figured she had a better place to be, said her goodbyes and when it got rough was happy to drift away on a cloud of morphine. It's an individual decision based on your age, your condition, your attitude. Chemo is definitely not for everyone.

Surprisingly, you can find doctors on the Internet urging you not to take the recommended poisons, to try alternative methods instead. Rare, but they're out there.

I questioned Sandi while we were jogging. Might I be a candidate for skipping chemo and go the dietary with meditation and herb route? She puffed out a resounding "Absolutely not!" Knowing ultimately it was my choice, she still expressed horror that I might think about chancing it "all naturally." She was quite adamant with her advice. "You should look into the natural treatments as they may work for you in *conjunction* with the therapies we suggest, but chemo and radiation are the way to go." End of story.

Okay, the majority of professionals are very pro-poison. This made me feel foolish for even contemplating skipping the big guns like chemo and radiation.

But we're talking about a perpetually confused woman who can take hours to decide what to wear each day. "Hmm, the black, navy or taupe pants? Maybe I should wear a dress? This skirt might work. What about leggings and a long top?" How could I possibly make a death-defying decision between chemotherapy and an alternative route? Wasn't this a question for my mother to decide?

It was starting to get frustrating; I don't do worrying or waiting well. It's an ADD thing called *patience non-existo*. You should see me in a lineup for a movie that has already started. I go berserk! My skin crawls and my heart races and I think I will die if I don't get inside the theater *this instant*. It's all I can do not to push the people in front of me. If it's an Old Dearie holding up the process with her walker and penny counting I calm down a little but still . . . Beep, beep! Get going, Grandma! You're not the only one that might not live long enough to see this show!

My four-week post-surgery date, the mandatory time out before receiving any other treatment, was October 12. I had healed nicely from the second surgery and was back to three-quarter speed with my life. I was over-ready to get the rest of this show on the road. Still I faced an extra three weeks of nail biting and (sugar-free) chocolate bingeing before my oncology consult, when we would find out if chemotherapy would be suggested or not. And we still hadn't heard if the consult would be conducted face to face in Kelowna or in front of a television set at the Community Cancer Services unit in Smithers.

At first the Kelowna receptionist told me video conferencing between Smithers and Kelowna couldn't be done, that they did not do video conferencing past Williams Lake, which is quite a ways south of us. I assured her the Smithers cancer unit had done it before with other BCCA centres. She only needed to get the oncologist on board to proceed. Then our techs could talk to her techs and do their thing.

She would have to get back to us.

Of course, it's all relative. It seems to take a long time but, in reality, things do move fairly quickly. I couldn't believe how fast I was processed for both surgeries. No time for weeks of mulling things over. Not like with knee injuries when your chances of getting a seat at the surgeon's office is right up there with scoring one of those $74 last-minute plane tickets to Mexico.

Still, I felt like I was inside a slowly digesting boa constrictor. This was *cancer.* You couldn't get it out of me or begin the treatment plan fast enough. Come on, people. Let's get this show on the road! Honk, honk!

Instead of road rage, cancer patients call it "staging rage." Staging is what a patient *needs* to have in hand before moving to the next phase in their battle. Surgical excision of your cancer does not mean you're done. Not by a long shot. What if they missed even one iota of a shred of a tentacle, an atom of cancerous dust which even now could be spreading via your blood? It's why they don't stop fighting after surgery. The war is not over.

Staging is a process whereby the severity of your cancer — the size, type and aggression level — is assessed. Knowing the state of the disease helps the doctor plan an appropriate treatment, meaning the weapons to continue the battle.

What *was* the holdup? Beep, BEEP!!! We had the results, we knew where the cancer was, where it wanted to be. Let's get our numbers together and see what else we're going to do to make sure I remained a living, breathing wife, mother, sister and friend.

Breast cancer staging is based on the range of the tumour (T), the degree of spread to the lymph nodes (N), and the indication of spreading to other body parts, called metastases (M).

(For an excellent chart on this, see the National Comprehensive Cancer Network's staging guide at www.nccn.com/understanding-cancer/cancer-staging.html)

A patient labelled "Tis" has a tumour "in situ," a carcinoma that has not spread to other tissue. That's a better stage than a T1–T4, which labels the size and extent of the tumour. The larger the number, the larger the problem.

Same with the lymph nodes. If there is no involvement, it's labelled "N0." The extent of the node involvement ranges from N1–N4, with N4 being the winner in a bad way. And with a metastasis, it's either a M0 (none) or M1.

Once the T, N, and M are determined, an overall "stage" of I, II, III, IV is assigned. These stages can also be split, using letters such as IIIA and IIIB.

It will turn out that I am T1N1M0 — tumour under 2 centimetres, one node positive and no distant metastasis. This translates as Stage IIA breast cancer, much less scary than anything with the number IV in it.

On October 19 the Kelowna Oncology department gave the thumbs-up for the video consult, saving us $1000 in expenses and two numb bums from 24 hours of watching scenery go by the window.

If I was sentenced to chemo, I could stay home, getting the drugs at the Smithers hospital. If there was to be no chemo, I had an appointment already booked for November 3rd in Kelowna with the radiation oncologist, so there wouldn't be much of a wait to get the radiation end of things going either. What a relief!

The best news was that somewhere in the kafuffle the oncology consult date changed from November 2 to October 22! Someone managed to save me 11 days of restless anxiety and downright childish moping. We would soon know what came next, how long I would be doing it for and what would happen while I was doing it. I would be able to map and plan some things for a change. Sort of like normal people did.

While marking the new dates on my calendar I noted a scrawl about an open women's cancer meeting being held in Smithers at

7 p.m. the following evening. I had been trying to attend one of those meetings for the past two months but the dates always conflicted with something.

On Wednesday night I carefully dressed in comfortable jeans and the cheeriest top I could find. On the 40-minute drive I wondered what I might ask of these women. What did I need to know about? I gathered my thoughts, feeling slightly intimidated about the whole thing for some reason. I get nervous around female strangers. They can be cruel and, while I doubted I would encounter such a thing in this setting, I wasn't sure I could handle it.

I'm the girl in Grade 6 who raised her hand, asking, "But how does the sperm get to the egg?" I brought down the house with that one. Seems you should know that by the time you're 11? The feeling of embarrassment over a simple, naïve question has haunted me ever since. I didn't want it to happen on this night. I definitely wouldn't be asking, "But how did the cancer get to the boob?"

It's a girl thing. We're so bad when it comes to worrying what others might think. Don't believe me? Ask a woman whom she dresses for when attending a party. The honest answer isn't always for her spouse and rarely for her; it's for the other women. They're the ones to be concerned about. They will suck in every inch of you and make on-the-spot judgments. "Oh my, Deb's put on weight. Isn't that dress a little short for her age? What is she trying to say with that hair colour? Tsk. Tsk. She must be having a tough go of things. The poor dear. Don't look at her . . . no, no! Don't look! She will think we're talking about her."

Some days I'm embarrassed to be labeled one and could almost hate other women. They can be daunting and unpredictable. Blinded by optimism, I don't see the punches coming until I'm flattened. Maybe I'd missed a class in grade school on plotting and scheming? It appears to be second nature to so many. Not my good friends, of course. That's why we're *friends*.

Really, I had nothing to worry about. It's not like I was faking anything or was a lookie-loo just being curious. I was a bona fide cancer fighter with scars to prove it. I belonged. I held an invisible cancer card, better than any credit card, which would get me through doors and out of chores when I wanted. So I took a deep breath and walked into the little office off Main Street. I said hello to two women milling about and glued myself beside a table full of books with a big donation jar sitting at one end. I put a $20 bill in and a woman moseyed over to thank me, handing me a pink rubber wristband with the breast cancer ribbon symbol and some writing on it. I put it around my wrist, thanking her as I did. The imaginary ice was broken.

Before long there were five of us seated in a circle, steaming mugs of herbal tea in hand. I had brought baked cookies and found there were some already provided. I ate one of theirs instead of mine. I didn't care if it was made with sugar or butter. I had a small hope it might be laced with marijuana. It's a known fact that cancer patients can get marijuana, or a derivative thereof, prescribed for pain in Canada. It would be an interesting way to spice up the gathering, although chances were I would end up scarfing all the baked goods before crawling under a table and falling asleep.

We introduced ourselves one at a time before expanding on what type of cancer we had and what treatment we would be having, had already had, or were going through. We talked about everything, no holds barred. I tried to grasp every word, asking for clarification when someone used a slang term or abbreviation I didn't know.

Attendance was mixed — mainly breast cancer survivors, a woman with a stomach tumour, and another with a husband who was having treatments for pancreatic cancer. But the one thing we all had in common was the need to talk about it. I didn't think I would ever shut up once it was my turn — maybe there *was* something in that cookie — but the others listened attentively, appreciating what had happened and filling me in on what was ahead.

One young woman wearing a wig had received her second round

of chemo. She looked pale, with dark circles beneath her eyes. Just like in the movies, I thought. OMG. Would that be me in a few months? She seemed rather blasé about what was happening to her, answering questions in short sentences, but telling us what we needed to know — how to balance your real life with your cancer life.

"You just keep going," she said.

I thanked her personally for coming to the meeting. "People like me need to talk to people like you, so thanks."

"Yeah, good luck," she said, her face slowly working itself into a smile. "Don't forget to buy Popsicles if you're going to get the chemo."

"Any flavour work better than others?" I asked.

"The margarita-flavoured ones."

It was so reassuring to see that life didn't end with chemo and that people on it could still muster up a smile and a joke. Wigged women are warriors, saints, heroes. I had needed to hear what was coming down the pipe first-hand and I got what I'd come for. I could feel the layers of fear stripping away as I read, talked and learned about cancer and the upcoming treatments. I drove home that night a little less anxious and for the first time in months, I slept right through the night.

Many communities have Canadian Cancer Society (CCS) volunteers who hold weekly or monthly meetings where you can sit and chat with other women who are in the process of beating breast cancer or have come out the other end. The CCS also has a service called Cancer Connection (1-888-939-3333) where you can call to talk to someone who has gone through whatever it is you are facing. Experienced volunteers sign up as contacts and you are welcome to ask them anything you need to know. It's free and it takes a load off your mind. You might make yourself a new friend right on the spot.

October 22 finally showed up on the calendar. All the guessing and thinking and worrying and wondering was about to end. Barry and I drove to Smithers without exchanging more than a few words. My mouth was dry, my armpits were soaked and I felt like I should be calling out "Dead woman walking" as we made our way to the cancer unit on the hospital's second floor. The chemo decision hung like a stone around my neck.

I was honoured with some pretty impressive support for my Consult Posse — my husband, who disguises himself as a retired pharmacist during the day; Sandi, my B&B doctor; and Dr. Z, a GP oncologist who works out of the Smithers cancer unit. We called her our go-to gal as she was the closest thing we had to a cancer specialist. They all sat with me in a tiny room usually used for counselling or wig modeling.

We fixated on the 36-inch TV screen when a cheery, petite woman with glasses came into view, seated herself at a desk and began talking. Dr. KJ reviewed my chart to make sure she understood everything correctly. There wasn't room for error here. We listened intently, most of us making notes. She asked me multiple health questions, including "Was there any cancer in the family?" I had to recount my menses and childbearing history for her and admit I had a pack-a-day habit for 21 years before quitting 13 years previously.

I would give anything if I could change that but quitting smoking was one of the hardest things I had ever done. It took five years of trying to quit before finally accomplishing it. The secret? You just stop. You tell yourself you will never go through the pain of withdrawal again if you never have another puff. Then you believe in that. Before you know it, the wanting-to-die phase ends and your days get easier.

After 13 years of being tobacco-free I figured I was out of the cancer woods. Now all these questions about it? Should we blame it on the cigarettes? Is that where this was going?

I squirmed in my chair. I had already answered many of these questions on numerous questionnaires for the surgeon's office, in the MRI department, on the colonoscopy paper work, even for ICBC after a recent motor vehicle accident. Who doesn't know that I had sex for the first time at age 17? Please raise your hand.

I hope you're not putting me into a category, Dr. KJ?

Oh, no, of course not, dear, but let's see, you smoked, drank, were promiscuous, and you've been known to cuss worse than Ozzy Osbourne. Of course you have cancer! You are a very bad, bad girl.

I felt the tears welling.

I'm not a bad girl, I'm not. I'm just . . . I'm just a person who has lived a little recklessly. I can change. I will change.

A tear ran down my face. I caught it mid roll and flicked it away.

None of that! No feeling sorry for yourself here. This is Judgment Day. Are you even listening to what's being said anymore?

Dr. KJ took a moment before summing up her prognosis.

She leaned across the desk, closer to the camera. The four of us automatically did the same from our end. It was so quiet you could have heard a fly breathing.

Here it was. The moment we had been waiting for. Drum roll, please . . .

I was told that because breast cancer did not run in my family and because it was a *micro* metastasis that it would be up to me to decide if I wanted chemo even though it had spread to one lymph node. I could either go with the chemo or bypass it and head straight to Kelowna for the radiation therapy.

I exhaled loudly, not realizing I'd been holding my breath. Wow! Knock me down with a grin! It was the PASS I had prayed for — no vile toxins, no nausea and vomiting, no compromised bone marrow, no infections, no losing my bloody hair! I felt light, like I could float around the room. Oh joy!

It took a second to realize the room was once again very, very quiet, that I was the only one smiling, like I just got an A on a paper that should have been marked D. It was obvious no one else had hoped for this. I realize now I had unconsciously made up my mind to skip the chemo if I could. I was that frightened of it.

My team was ready though and threw a hard ball. They asked to hear "the numbers."

Wait, no, I don't need to hear the statistics, do I? Wouldn't it be like listening to my husband's stock channel? Would it really make a difference? Would other people's decisions have anything at all to do with mine? I didn't have to do this if I didn't want to, right? (Was that a touch of spoiled snotty-talk, there?)

It didn't matter. No one heard what I answered because three other voices overrode mine.

"Yes, let's hear the numbers."

I didn't absorb them but the bottom line was this: chances of a recurrence dropped significantly if I did the chemo and the possibility of a repeat surgery practically disappeared. My insecurities would stay small instead of growing into something that ate my brains out over the next five years.

I didn't want to listen but ultimately it was my choice and I needed to make an informed decision, not one based on fear. I would be on "the lightest protocol" but still it would be two drugs strong enough to kill hair follicles, fingernails and cancer cells. They wanted to put Mr. Clean through my veins.

I remember feeling a bit swoonish at that. I pictured the possessed Linda Blair at her worst. Green skin, cracked nails and black lips. Maybe she hadn't been possessed? Just had a bad chemo reaction?

The tie-breaker was Dr. Z asking me if I could live with myself if, years down the road, I had a recurrence and had turned down the chemo. Aw crap. That got to me. She was right. I would need to be able to tell myself I did everything I could to make sure those cancer cooties never took me down again. I needed to buck up and start fighting. Holing up in a lymph node! That was just plain nasty. It was time to take my body back once and for all.

Cue the *Rocky* theme song.

While all this rolled around in my head, Dr. Z asked Barry a question. Was I comfortable taking risks or would I forever worry about ducking the harder path? Or something to that effect.

Barry didn't even pause. I think his exact words were "She will go insane."

I had to agree. I would be an absolute rubber room candidate if I didn't agree to the chemo. Then, if the cancer did come back, I wouldn't be blaming myself. I would blame my husband; he was the next in line. Before the conference ended I had decided it would be a winter without hair.

7

Prepping for the Vein Drano

My next appointment was for blood work, which was done at the Health Centre in Houston. It was to make sure I was healthy enough to withstand the upcoming treatments. I also had a physical with Sandi. Heart and lungs, check. Eyes, ears, nose and mouth, check. Attitude: changed to optimistic. All vital systems go for chemo.

Later that day I drove to Smithers for another eye-widening discussion with Alice at the cancer unit. Alice would be administering the chemo, and she explained to me exactly what would be happening, right down to what and what not to eat on the day of a treatment. I was given a yellow folder this time. Inside were info sheets on my two chemo drugs, their side effects, and how to deal with vomiting and diarrhea, sore gums, heartburn, and taste changes.

I also completed a medications sheet with Alice to help me remember what anti-nausea pills — dexamethasone and ondansetron — to take, and when, before I came for the intravenous chemotherapy drugs, cyclophosphamide and docetaxel.

It was very confusing at first.

The info sheets boldly announced that "alcohol does not appear to affect the safety or usefulness of the anti-nauseate." Think maybe it was the number one question from cancer patients? So no, you don't have to be abstemious in order to get through this. Common sense tells me that my body would already be overwrought with the offensive chemicals. Why kick it when it was down?

There would be four treatments with three weeks spread between each. The entire ordeal would take another 12 weeks out of my life. A whole trimester of the unknown, like being pregnant, and I managed to get through that twice, I reminded myself.

They say people continue to work and do chemotherapy. Well, if they could do this then so could I. A surgeon in Vernon once told me I "came from good stock." I intended to continue proving him right. I could do this! Easy, peasie. I had gone without chocolate that long. I think. Possibly. Okay, I probably hadn't. But I was an aerial photographer for three months once. I used to go green every time we went up in the tiny two-seater airplane. If the pilot hadn't continually tried to make me sick to win a bet with his buddies, I might have made it to the four-month mark. I would like to say I puked in his lap before quitting but no such luck. I simply walked away on tottering legs to a better-paying job on the terra firma.

This was going to be tougher than that, Alice said, but assured me I had made the right decision. I barely listened, still reeling from being so close to the escape door and not taking it.

What had I set in motion *this* time?

Part of the "cancer care package" got me a free visit to a nutritionist and a counsellor. The latter was in Prince George, so I probably wouldn't make the seven-hour round trip to lie on a couch and moan about my husband enjoying his wine while I was abstaining. But I did take advantage of the nutritionist.

I sat before this newest professional in full blame mode. Eyes down, head hung, ready to hit myself if she just said the word. Shame on me. I caused this cancer to happen by my own stupidity: the alcohol, the chocolate, the ice cream and cookies.

But no . . . we go over my usual diet, finding room for improvement in a few departments. More fruit and water. Less red meat, even if it is organic. Together we agree smoothies made with strawberries and sugarless, fat-free yogurt would be much healthier than a jumbo bag of licorice. She assured me I was on the right path with my resolve to cut the drinking down to the three to five a week and said there wasn't an actual anti-cancer diet that she could give me. She did steer me to some books, one called *A Dietitian's Cancer Story: Information & Inspiration for Recovery & Healing* by D. Dyer and the other called *Cancer Survivor's Nutrition & Health Guide: Eating Well and Getting Better During and After Cancer Treatment* by G. Spiller and B. Bruce.

In seeking knowledge through literary sources I devoured a library of books on cancer. I Googled and Yahooed, spending hours long into the night trying to track down any recommended miracle cures to stop the spread of the disease to other parts of my body. A surgeon had cut it out but was it 100 percent gone? There were slim margins that it wasn't. That's why the chemo and the radiation, yet surely there was something I could do to help?

Before long, I had multiple notebooks with long lists of weird plant concoctions and "panic" remedies. In the beginning there was a phase of wanting to take anything that would prevent this nightmare from ever occurring again. I would have rolled in snake oil, choked down dried kangaroo dung or smeared lizard guts over my breast had I thought it would help.

It all became so confusing. Never mind the shaman rituals and all the holistic ventures. I needed to focus on what supplements and vitamins and foods I should be pumping into myself to prepare for the upcoming onslaught. Yet even that became a swirling jumble of advice from 50 different directions. For example, I read: Take L-glutamine when you're on chemotherapy. L-glutamine is the most abundant free-form amino acid in the body and is very important for maintaining gastrointestinal and stimulated immune cell functioning. It is an important transporter of nitrogen (and carbon) in the body and therefore is vital in wound healing.

I also read L-glutamine may increase the effectiveness of some forms of chemotherapy but it *may also stimulate tumour growth*. Doctors are very cautious about recommending anything that is not officially FDA-approved for treatment. Although there were numerous studies "proving" the benefits of the supplement, L-glutamine does not have the official FDA approval and therefore should not be prescribed or recommended.

Who do you believe? The last thing I wanted was to promote more tumour growth or impede the cleanup drugs. Why put myself through that and then hamper the results? I had to admit it sounded exactly like something I would do.

After talking with Dr. Z at the Smithers cancer unit, I decided to turn to a naturopath for additional advice on diet and vitamins. The info sheets I received from Alice in the yellow folder had helpful, detailed instructions on what to eat for upset stomach and other ailments. There was nothing on supplements to help protect your organs while the "Drano" was plunged through. For the price of $200, the naturopath straightened out the muddle. He advised me on which vitamins and concoctions would fortify my body, the armour to protect my good things while the chemo was kicking some serious cancer butt!

We talked for close to two hours, my hand getting writer's cramp near the end. We discussed the before, during and after regime. The chemo supplements were different from what I should take during the radiation treatments. Then I wrote a page on what I should do for the rest of my life.

As a rare health food patron, I spent the good part of an hour in the Smithers store trying to figure out what I was looking for. Quinoa? Q10? Propolis? Where did one start to clean up their life? Three hundred dollars later I came out of the store, armed and dangerous. It was going to be a massacre and I was going to triumph. Of that, I was pretty certain. Mostly. Some. Pass me the organic 85 percent chocolate, please.

Speaking of eating, there had been plenty of discussion on the chemo's side effects . . . like nausea, constipation (or the opposite), and how it was going to make things taste different. I would probably experience a very dry mouth, perhaps with sores. Seeing my dentist before starting the chemo was highly recommended. Chemo would compromise the immune system so infections needed to be dealt with first. It was also suggested I purchase alcohol-free mouthwash, Biotene dry-mouth toothpaste and the softest toothbrush I could find. I did all of the above and was thankful for it. A supply of fruit Popsicles in your freezer (*Should I make some with lime and tequila?* I wondered. *Did that stuff even freeze?*) and ice-cold sports drinks were mentioned as well.

What did people do if they couldn't afford all this stuff? Good grief. List that as another side effect — guilt over going through this as a pampered diva and not like the thousands who simply tough it out. No gold credit card, no glorious support line . . . just someone with a malignant growth inside that's trying to steal their life.

And then there was my mental health. I had been so busy getting my physical self ready I hadn't spent much time preparing mentally. If I was going to get through this I would need to overcome the fear of all the horrible things I imagined chemo to be. I made myself up a mantra to repeat in case things got really bad.

I asked for these drugs because I believe in them.

Repeat.

I asked for these drugs because I believe in them.

Okay, so I was not quite there yet. Repeating this made my nose sniffly and my eyes blurry. Maybe if I sang the mantra to the tune of something funny? What was comical enough to override a chemo mantra?

"Never laugh when a hearse goes by, 'cause you may be the next one to die . . . harrumph, harrumph . . ."

I am hopeless.

On a brisk November 2nd I travelled to the Smithers cancer unit to meet with Alice again. We were becoming friends and I always looked forward to seeing her. Despite her job of caring for the sick and dying, Alice managed a genuine smile for everyone and I felt instantly calm in her presence. Not many people have that effect on me.

I was there because of some confusion with my treatment protocol. Turns out one of my drugs would be changed and Alice needed to review side effects with me — stuff like my nails possibly getting thick and black, and falling off. I was in stitches laughing. "Where do you people get this stuff?" I asked. Are my boobs going to explode? Would my eyes start flashing like turn signals on a car? This was so not funny.

Was that hysteria I heard in that cackle? Wasn't this where someone was supposed to slap me and yell, "Get hold of yourself"?

I asked for these drugs because I believe in them.

I asked for these drugs because I believe in them.

Are you frickin' kidding me? Run, Deb. Run for the hills.

After my fun with Alice, I had an appointment to see a registered massage therapist (RMT) who specializes in lymphatic drainage. The amusement just never ended. Most women with breast cancer have two types of surgery — a lumpectomy or a mastectomy, to get rid of the tumour, and an axillary dissection to remove underarm lymph nodes. The body's lymphatic drainage system gets rid of waste products from the normal functioning of cells. I had a total of 12 lymph nodes extracted, which meant my waste disposal system was compromised, putting me at risk for lymphedema. Lymphedema is swelling caused by backed-up lymphatic fluid, sort of like the reservoir behind a dam. The result can be a painful, swollen arm on the affected side.

A newly formed cave beneath my armpit attested to the surgeon's diligent mining technique. The scar from the axillary node surgery ran horizontally across my side, almost directly beneath the armpit. The scar tissue was an angry-looking pink, meaning it was busy trying to heal. The surgical scars around my nipple had settled down into a faint brownish line. Barely noticeable. What *was* noticeable was the off-kilter headlight alteration where my nipple pointed right instead of straight ahead. Still, I thought I could get *some* appreciation at a wet T-shirt contest. Not that I'd been in one in the past 25 years, but that thought never goes away. I'm still 30-something, aren't I?

Tamara, the Smithers RMT, was impressed I could already bend my elbow back behind my head. The stretch felt fantastic. A measuring tape appeared and my measurements were taken in four separate places along my arm for the record. Ideally, I should have had her take my measurements before surgery so we would have a baseline arm circumference, but I didn't. It was easy to talk myself out of it as it costs close to $90 for a visit to an RMT. I was already paying that for treatments to correct whiplash suffered in a car accident a year earlier. The soft tissue damage in my upper left back still plagued me. We didn't have extended medical. So okay, I cheaped out. Never mind my money being siphoned off at an alarming rate by the health food store. Something had to give, and arm circumference measurements took the hit.

Why doesn't somebody just shake me sometime? This was my health we were talking about. Maybe a few less chai tea lattes, eh Deb?

As Tamara massaged the axillary scar area with her fingertips, pulling and stretching the skin away from the scar to free up the movement, she told me more about lymph node drainage; how it worked with the rest of the body to dispose of debris and microorganisms that can cause infection and how to prevent blockages. Lymphedema is a scary thing and sometimes it can't be reversed. You're stuck with a swollen limb, which is fine if you're a tree or a male gigolo.

A thicker or engorged feeling would be a sure sign I needed to either get in to a registered massage therapist or try and drain it myself. There are a few ways to do this. Tamara showed me how to use my left hand to apply slight pressure on my skin and pat in a fast sweeping motion against the skin, petting and drawing it toward my core. She drew arrows on my skin with an erasable marker so that I could remember the next day which way to sweep up or down the arm or under the armpit. It is a light motion but should be done for 10 minutes, which tired my good arm. Plan B, she said, would be swimming laps for 10 minutes or jumping on a rebounder or trampoline for as long. I added "mini rebounder" to my Dear Santa wish list.

Lack of funds or not, I did have to return to a RMT two weeks after this initial visit. In reality, even though it can be painful as they stretch and pull at tender skin, it always helped more than it hurt. The range of mobility before and after a visit was impressive. But that's not why I went. Robyn, an enthusiastic young RMT, came to Houston once a week. I gave her a call after developing some alarming roping down my midriff. It felt like an old-fashioned telephone cord was beneath my skin. You could see the lines bulging along my torso. It began beneath my right breast and spiraled down to just slightly above my navel. There were four of them side-by-side. I couldn't stop running my hand over them. They were out-of-this-world bizarre.

This phenomenon happens to 50 percent of women who have had axillary dissection, and it can develop in your wrist, up your arm or start as high as your armpit. Or, as in my case, on your abdomen. They are hardened lymphatic vessels which have been altered by the surgery. They often rupture on their own within a few weeks. But I didn't want to wait for fear they would get worse.

Robyn knew just what to do and started pulling the area with one hand while pushing with the other. Before long we heard a "snap" and looked at each other with a grin. Success. One cord was broken. It took close to 30 minutes to get the rest to break, none of which caused any pain. Once that happened, the cords relaxed and faded away. We were free to concentrate the rest of the hour on that sore back of mine. Ahhh. Nothing beat a good massage.

Another good thing happened in my life at this time. My regular dentist opened his practice to share patients with his brother-in-law, Dr. Yummy, as women in the Bulkley Valley named him. Bar none, Dr. Yummy is the most attractive man I have ever laid eyes on.

If we're to be totally honest here, which I have been up to now, then I have to talk about the first time I saw Dr. Y. It was one of those intense moments, the frozen-in-time kind you never forget — the first step on the moon's surface, the day Diana died and the minute my eyes settled on this much younger, extremely hot foreigner.

Here I was, an older woman sprinting toward my 50s like there was a race. A woman who loves her husband even after 20 years of him going right and her left, of bickering about the way each other drives, parks, eats, talks, fill-in-the-blanks . . . all balanced by realizing the value of the years invested in each other, shared memories, the families, the understanding that one likes champagne and orange juice in the morning and the other protein powder. And we still sizzle, if you know what I mean. In short, I was not, and never had been, in the market for a replacement. My hands were full with the man I had.

I was at the dentist's office not because I had a sore tooth but because it was on the pre-chemo to-do list. And that is why I was leaning on the ledge above receptionist Sheryl's desk, talking to her about the local ski hill. We were both looking forward to opening day in another month. The door to the examining room opened and out walked Dr. Y.

He was lofty but not gangly, with a smallish waist and a full chest rising to wide shoulders. The word would be "adventurously" handsome with brown hair and eyebrows dark enough to border on black. His even white teeth contrasted finely against his tanned skin, suggesting he spent a lot of time outdoors. Dr. Y was wearing a thin blue T-shirt that adorned his frame like dressing on a salad.

I grabbed Sheryl's elbow. "Who is that?" I whispered, my eyes never leaving him as he strode across the hall into my usual dentist's office.

"That's your new dentist." Her thinly disguised grin revealed she enjoyed delivering this news. It was obvious I wasn't the first to have such a reaction.

"No," I whispered. "No, no. He's too cute."

The well-proportioned, tanned man came out of the office and returned to the examining room, closing the door behind him but not before turning and flashing a broad smile in my direction.

Did that just happen? For a second, the world stopped turning. My heart skipped a dozen beats then took off like it was being chased.

"He's sharing the practice with his brother-in-law."

My eyes squinted. "Sharing? What exactly does that mean?"

I recall my voice was rather high-pitched and squeaky.

"It means you get who you get when you come. That's okay with you, isn't it?"

Oh, she was enjoying this to the max. She knew exactly how I was feeling. Like a doe-eyed 15-year-old, albeit a doe with crow's feet and facial fault lines deep enough to fall into.

"So this man is married to Dr. L's sister?"

Did it matter?

"Other way around. Dr. L is married to Dr. Y's sister. Dr. Y is single."

There was that grin again.

I wanted to scream, "I am not interested." I was happy with my life the way it was. Who would want to think about putting another man into it? Okay, I couldn't help it if my body didn't understand this and was responding energetically to the visual stimuli. It responded the same way to butter-fried onions at a hot dog stand but, I am proud to say, I can enjoy the fragrance and walk on by.

Really. Was this a bad thing? I mean, honestly. What harm could this be other than having to sit with an erratic heartbeat for a 30-minute visit? I could handle it. Maybe this would be a nice thing. What did I have against sitting in the same room with a man who looked like he could cause a stampede of high heels with one blink of those long eyelashes? Was I getting that old, unable to appreciate a work of art when I saw one? To stop and smell the roses when they were near? To melt into a puddle at the feet of . . .

The door to the exam room opened again and out walked a young woman wearing a frozen, lop-sided smile and the same glazed expression I'm sure I wore. Who wouldn't fall for this guy? I took a deep breath and decided to enjoy this. I looked to the ceiling in what was as close to a prayer as I get these days. *Oh, karma,* I said, *I must have done something very right in my life to deserve this.*

And that thought led me to the next one.

"Mother," I murmured gratefully under my breath. Of course! This made sense now. The treat of meeting someone so dazzling was something she would try and send to me from the other side and I bet she'd found a way. My mom would do anything to cheer up her loved ones. She must have known I needed a boost. (This is the ADD mind in full swing. We might fail in many departments, but imagination isn't one of them.)

I was shown into the examination room. The door closed behind Sheryl but not before I received a discreet wink. That set me even further on edge. I get nervous talking to the intercom at the drive-thru, never mind facing a Hollywood dreamboat in a 20-square-foot cubicle. To talk about *me*! And when I get nervous, I never know what will fall out of my mouth.

I was on high alert. The door swung wide and in he came. His eyebrows arched with his easy smile and it was as if someone poked me with a hot stick. I leaped from my seat, hand outstretched.

"Hi. My name is Deb Smith, I don't believe we've met," I said, like I was at a cocktail party or something. His smile widened and we parted, backing into our respective places. I lay back on the inclined dental chair, feeling like I was in a shrink's office.

Ever hear of nervous chatter? With me it's more like a cork coming out of a champagne bottle. I talk fast and without focus, skipping from one thought to another, from A to F, to B to K and back to the beginning again. I repeat myself, flick my eyes around the room and drool. Probably. I'm not sure about that last one, but I do everything else, so I can't be sure.

I talked about my mother, my worries and my life. I opened up like a liquid book and poured myself out all over the room. He watched my face intently, listening to every syllable. He asked me questions and then went to get the X-ray technician to take pictures of my teeth.

I didn't really hear what Dr. Y said. My heart was making too much noise. They shouldn't let men that handsome be professionals. How could anyone pay attention? Heaven forbid I should need to hear something really important from him. I actually remember thinking that. What I don't remember is leaving. I think I floated out to my vehicle.

Yes, I told Barry about it and was teased relentlessly for the next month. I tell *you* all this because it prepares you for a story yet to unfold. Patience, please.

Next on the pre-chemo checklist was a flu shot. Highly, highly recommended. I had never had a flu shot before because almost everyone I knew who did got sick. Seemed counterproductive to me. But it was expounded that a flu shot was only an inoculation for certain types of extra-dastardly flu bugs that were circulating at the time. It couldn't possibly cover all the types of flu I might get exposed to, but it would help fortify me against the most dangerous ones. Oh, okay. Sign me up.

Luckily, flu shot clinics were happening in Smithers, so back I went to get in line with 30 other shot seekers. We flashed our B.C. Medicare cards before filling out a questionnaire and taking a seat to wait for our names to be called.

I was given a very timely gift last Christmas by my children who were concerned about their mother's increasing forgetfulness. It was a portable Nintendo game player into which you could insert different games. The ones they sent were called Brain Age, quick questions of addition, multiplication, etc. that forced your brain to work. A picture of an airplane taking off appeared when you were jet quick. When you weren't the turtle icon appeared. It seemed to help. So far I hadn't forgotten any of my kid's names.

The games made waiting room lineups disappear. I was always absorbed in the middle of a game when my name was called. What? Already?

Back at the flu clinic there was a quick "Owww!" and it was over. I was officially inoculated against *some* strains of the flu. I half expected a bold *S* to appear on my chest, like Superman. Bring on the kryptonite.

8

Chemo Exposed: The Raw Details

My friends figure I'm a feet-first, jump-into-anything kind of girl. Yes, I could be impulsive, but when it came to parties, travelling or chemo sessions, I leave nothing to chance. That's why the night before my first chemo session rolled around I was a loaded spring. My checklist had ticks beside every item — Popsicles, gum, soft toothbrush, dry-mouth toothpaste and mouthwash, vitamins, electric razor and a fridge filled with healthy foods. It was like the first day of school with a shiny lunchbox, scribblers, pencils, erasers, new outfit . . .

Whoa! Back up! New outfit? What would I wear to my first chemo session? Alice and I had never discussed it. Was there a dress code? Like pajamas and housecoat? Too casual was just not me, especially for such an important moment. What about all black, to symbolize having cancer, juxtaposed with my celebratory 50th-year tiara? Wearing my tiara never failed to make me feel better. That's why I've bought one for most of my friends, so they can feel wonderful at special times, too. It was only after a hard second thought that I decided a tiara might be considered excessive. Honestly, I kid you not.

Deep down, I was a cyclonic neurotic stressing about everything but the big picture. My mind churned with the problem. Polyester anything was out in case I got a chill, but then wait . . . I might get hot flashes, they said, so poly might be nice. Maybe start with the basics. Get out the good bra in case I got too hot, too fast; some big girl panties, of course. Don't forget those!

I decided on a light blue sweater of my mom's that made my grey eyes look brighter. It would be comforting having something of my mother's with me. It was one of her favourite Talbots sweaters. Add comfy stretch-corduroy jeans and a neck scarf in case I bled or puked or . . . ? A thousand horrors flicked through my mind. A wide scarf perhaps.

The following morning I was exhausted but hyper, having slept poorly due to the anti-nausea steroids. I must have run four miles inside the house looking for items I had set down. My keys, my iPod, my keys again. Sharon arrived a bit early, knowing I would be fretting. She was the friend I ran to after discovering I might need the chemo so I figured it fitting that she accompany me to the first session. Sharon was a nurse who left her calling to become mayor of Houston for eight years. Having her with me for such a huge ordeal meant a lot.

What *about* Barry?

Well, after much consideration, I didn't think a chemo room would be the best place for my husband. Barry has the uncanny ability to say exactly the wrong thing to me when I am at my lowest. I couldn't take the chance he might push my teetering mental state off its narrow ledge. I'd hate to get my first chemo in restraints.

So Sharon was my rock. I handed her the Suburban keys, too nervous to get behind the wheel myself.

"You look fine," she said after a quick glance at my attire.

(See? With Barry I had to extract compliments with a glass of Scotch and a pry bar.)

We made it to Smithers in good time, parked outside the hospital entrance and trundled up to the second-floor cancer unit lugging a bag packed with lunch and snacks, spare clothes (in case of any "accidents") and the stack of information sheets, books and pills I had been issued. Homer the bear was in his carry satchel and I held a rose, one of many Barry had given me the day before . . . something beautiful to focus on.

Look out, we're moving in!

The cancer unit staffers were kind enough not to laugh. I'm sure they had seen it all before, though not to this extreme.

My mad dash to the washroom produced only a nervous dribble. It would be the last time that happened as I was about to start drinking two liters of water a day to help flush the chemo toxins. I needed that much just to wash down the fistful of vitamins and supplements pills I had started taking.

I came out of the washroom and that's when I noticed it to my right. The Chemo Chair. My internal temperature spiked. I was on fire. I wanted to rip off all of my clothes and run down the hallway in search of a snow bank. I turned back to the washroom and splashed cold water on my face. My armpits were soaked. Sweat ran down my back.

"Alice, I'm having an attack of some kind," I yelled from inside the washroom, clutching the neckline on my sweater.

A smiling face appeared in the doorway.

"It's the steroids, it will pass."

"Are you sure? Look at the blotches on my face! I think I'm coming down with something?" Panic was gathering.

"Come out here," Alice called. "We have an electric fan."

I did as I was told and within minutes my internal meltdown started to subside. It was the first of many, many power surges to come.

I returned to the chemo area. Five La-Z-Boy chairs ringed the room, all facing a large window which held a panoramic view of the Hudson Bay Mountain ski runs. One of my favourite places in the entire world. I couldn't have asked for anything better.

I pushed myself backward into relaxed mode. A beautiful pre-heated quilt, made and donated by a former patient, was wrapped around me. Two Ativan pills (an anti-anxiety drug) were popped under my tongue. Before long I felt calm . . . *calm* . . . *calm* . . . and then I heard "The chemo drugs haven't arrived yet."

I bolted straight up in the chair.

WHAT! The chemo drugs haven't arrived? Does that mean we won't be doing this today?

My heart was racing, my palms pasty. *You mean I'll have to go through all this again?*

I could see Alice was on the phone.

"They're still in the hospital pharmacy and will be here in a few minutes."

My shoulders sagged in relief. *A few minutes . . . okay, calm down.* I closed my eyes and listened to the Mozart piece playing in the background.

"Look Deb, I can see fresh snow on the runs!"

(See why I brought Sharon along? My husband would have had me embroiled in an argument about the weather by now.)

Alice reappeared wearing a thick rubber apron tied over her hospital uniform, industrial strength rubber gloves tucked beneath her arm.

"The drugs are here," she said, looking very serious. A needle appeared out of nowhere.

Although I had big, clearly visible veins in my hand and wrist, getting the short, fine tube called a cannula into one of them proved problematic. Once the cannula is in and secured with tape it's connected to IV tubing through which the chemo is delivered into the bloodstream. But Alice had to get the needle in first. She tried a second vein. She was normally such a rock but you could see it caused her pain to think she was hurting me.

I told her it was fine. The Ativan was working. *Smile.* "T–a–k–e y–o–u–r t–i–m–e."

After a third attempt she called Loretta, another nurse, who also had trouble but finally got the IV in and working. No worries, I assured everyone. Dr. H in Terrace already won the Grimace Award for that pre-surgical wire placement. For that much pain, I should have left the hospital with a baby.

Sharon's fussing with my blankets and a surprise visit from Sandi, who had been downstairs working the emergency room all night, distracted me momentarily from the business at hand. But the needle was in, the bag of terror hooked to the IV pole and, though I tried hard not to notice, the drip started. The moment came, a tear loomed large and then I looked away.

And it was all fine. I did not feel anything, except relief. I had imagined a big surge of caustic stinging or burning or a metallic drip down my throat. But there was nothing so we returned to laughing and chatting.

I was doing this. Must be the big girl panties? I wasn't used to wearing them.

The 90 minutes passed so fast. I was amazed when the rubber-clad Alice returned to take the deflated bag down from the IV rack, flush my vein with saline, and hang the second bag of skull and crossbones.

For this one I had to wear frozen oven mitts to help stop the flow of drug into my hands. There was a chance it would affect the nails to the point where they thickened, blackened and possibly fell off. The mitts, I was assured, worked well. They were bulky and freezing. Goose bumps rose across my arms and Sharon tugged the quilt higher up my torso. So much for reading, game playing, eating or drinking. Next time I would arrive much lighter and less accessorized.

But what about my toenails? I worried. Not wanting the drug to circulate into my toes, I quickly ditched my warm shoes and tried keeping my feet up in the air as I asked the question. Barry and I had an unplanned plan to hit a beach somewhere if I got through all this. Would I have to go with black beans for toenails? Or worse, become one of those people ridiculed for wearing socks inside their sandals? I would ask for an ice foot bath next visit. I was a big believer in practicing prevention (right, this from the woman who has permanently disconnected the smoke alarm in the kitchen).

Two other patients had wandered in between my drug change. Closest to me was an elderly lady in a tightly curled brown wig. We exchanged pleasantries before she politely pretended to ignore our little party. To her right was a white-haired man looking relaxed behind a newspaper. *He must be a pro?* I thought.

I found out later the two of them had cancers that made my breast issues sound trivial. My four treatments seemed paltry stacked against their 20-plus. I was an impostor surrounded by friends, a rose and a stuffed bear. What planet was I even from? Good thing I left my tiara home.

It was over before we were ready . . . three hours and one hospital meal later. No time to run the movie we had brought. With all the questions and talking and eating and drinking, there hadn't been time to get nervous. A morning of distraction; they knew me so well! Although I'd come close, I'd survived without *totally* embarrassing myself. The next three treatments were going to be a breeze. Maybe I'd let Barry come for the next one? Now that I knew the routine the stress would be much less.

Sandi went home to sleep and Sharon and I went shopping.

What? Actually, I was surprised myself; amazed that I felt fine, still juiced from my jittery nerves and the steroids. There was energy there. We were in Smithers with the Christmas season looming. The good stuff moves fast in the few stores we have in the North so a post-chemo visit would have to work. I bumped into a few displays and counters but didn't break anything.

I made it for another hour before the crash that followed every high arrived. Sharon whisked me home, listening to me snore all the way. Once home I made it to the couch where I slept until 10 p.m. I awoke wondering which end was up. Was it morning or night and did I need to take a pill for anything? A little heartburn, a headache and dryness at the back of my throat led me to down half a Tylenol 3 tablet. Otherwise all was good. The chemo was in and it was staying in. I felt a flash of pride. Or was that another heat wave coming on?

On November 6, four days after administration of the docetaxel and cyclophosphamide, I figured a combination of food poisoning and alcohol poisoning at the same time would be a walk in the park compared to this. I felt like rank, polluted, low-grade crud.

There was a sheet of paper somewhere amidst all the piles of pages I'd been given that listed possible symptoms I might experience. No one mentioned the possibility I would get them *all*, and all at the same time. Where were the numbers of probability, here? Why hadn't I asked about those numbers before treatment . . . the percentage of losers that get everything but a hammer thrown at their head?

There was a thick coated feeling, almost numbness, inside of my mouth. The books labeled this "dry mouth." It was an accurate description, although "blinding sandstorm inside a dust bowl" was accurate as well. It made me want to nibble and chew on the inside walls of my mouth, which was probably why people developed mouth sores. There was a metallic, salty taste, like I had licked rust off someone's bumper. I had heartburn and achy knee joints and felt like I had aged 40 years. My head pounded in the front and on the sides. My hot flashes were so intense I thought I might drown in my own sweat.

Nothing tasted the way it should so I wandered around trying to rid my mouth of that awful sensation with things that just made it worse. My usual frozen raspberries were spit out along with the orange juice, the water, even chocolate milk! Go figure? There was a constant burn in the back of my throat and on top of it all, I felt like a tsunami-sized flu was coming down on top of my head. My stomach was in constant turmoil. I couldn't read, sit for a movie, or write a letter. I figured I would have to stop talking to people soon as I couldn't seem to say one single positive thing at the moment. And word was I had yet to hit bottom.

That happened between 7 and 10 p.m. when I wandered the house, hoping a plane would fall from the sky and squish me like a bug. I went from window to window searching the horizon. Being in my skin was painful.

I managed to swim for 40 minutes early on the first day but my resolve to exercise daily dragged itself right out the window the next morning. I would have to play this game by ear.

Same for doing this the low-cal way. I had stocked the fridge with low fat, no fat, sugar free and within four days I had been to the store twice to stock up on the groceries I was trying to avoid. I wanted mashed potatoes, buttered bread, canned mushroom soup, cheese sauce, cheese ravioli and a gallon of milk. All in the name of trying to put the fire out. I had planned on abstaining from dairy, wheat and sugar for the three months. What did I know? Why do I always figure I know what I am doing?

This was some kind of reality check . . . the world telling me I needed to change how I look at things. I plan on it being one way and when it isn't, I'm crushed and left floundering. Like I was feeling at the moment. Bewildered, worried about how much worse this could get and wondering how people got through it?

And the worst of it was, I would get through this, get stronger, and then have to do it again and again and again. It was emotionally devastating. A real-life joy sucker. I forced myself to think of the multitude of children who went through this. How could I be such a wuss when little kids experienced this hell? This type of thinking did nothing but sink my ship further.

After Tylenol for the sore joints, a heartburn tablet and an anti-nausea pill, I slept right through my fifth post-chemo night until nine in the morning. Barry checked on me twice, more than a little worried I was dead. I know I experienced a few flashes of intense heat and had sailed the bed covers far and wide more than twice during the night, but the heat waves didn't seem to disturb my rest like they had. Maybe this waned after the first few days?

My helpful husband put on his pharmacist cap and insisted I pop another anti-nausea pill and down the tall glass of Gatorade he had poured. Within minutes I felt not too bad for the first time in 48 hours. Good enough to get up and make a bowl of oatmeal and go for a walk in an amazing display of sunshine that was happening in the world beyond my windows. Tromping through the two inches of fresh snow was fun, although my knees still ached and I couldn't believe I was jogging only three days ago. I felt like an old woman with "jiddy joints," as Barry's Granny used to call them. He didn't realize dear old Granny was trying not to swear in front of a kid. I'm pretty sure she meant G.D. joints.

My attitude lightened even more with the discovery of things that helped settle my stomach, like Jell-O and those lime Popsicles (no tequila, I'm afraid), ice cream and hummus. Then there were the things I should definitely avoid like spices and metal utensils. And raspberries? For some reason my love of raspberries went south and I had to spit them out. I still can't eat a raspberry without tasting metal in my mouth.

"Whatever worked" was my new motto. I felt a small sense of excitement toward dinner that night. To heck with what the nutritionist said. I was planning on comfort food that wouldn't hurt my mouth. Everything felt so raw and tender in there. No toast, no tortilla chips, no crackers, no nuts for me.

I still had two more days before I hit my nadir, the lowest point in my immune system functioning during the three-week chemo cycle. I had to be careful of infection, avoiding large groups of people, crowded rooms, anyone with a cold.

Day 10 after the caustic juice, and I said thank goodness for make-up. My face, chest and back had broken out in acne. I had gone from being a woman who used only a slight wave of mascara and lipstick to a gal with a briefcase of cover-up and colouring products. The problem was I didn't know how to use them, to blend or co-ordinate or whatever it was those intimidating models in the cosmetic departments did. I ended up looking like a troubled clown with psychotic cosmetic issues.

Just quit looking in the mirror, I told myself. Tug, tug . . . the hair was still there, although my skull was tingling and I scratched it frequently. Sigh. It was still all good. I licked my numb lips. Well, mostly all good. The only thing that stood between chemo-me and the old-me resided mostly in my mouth. I kept biting and nibbling at the insides of it and there was an ache that went up into my ears. Nothing tasted right and I was thinking that issue was going to last the entire three months. Suddenly I loved Gatorade and tea with milk and honey!

They say days 7 to 10 are the bottom. So here we were and it wasn't bad at all. My energy was climbing back up, possibly from all the sweets I'd been allowing myself. The naturopath advised strongly against refined sugar during chemo as it feeds cancer cells. So I was trying to go with the maple syrup, honey, stevia-thing. "Tried" being the operative word. If they made sugarless, dark chocolate Kit Kats, I would have been okay.

The biggest concern was being constantly dehydrated, so much so I dropped five pounds — all liquid. You could see it. My breasts shrank two sizes and looked like long, skinny raisins instead of plump grapefruits. The sports drinks, even though they contained about 42 grams of sugar per bottle, helped counter the dehydration and that was a priority. Regular water tasted horrible, but I have since been told that adding lemon helps cut that metallic taste.

Barry purchased bottled water from every store in Houston . . . purified, osmosis processed, filtered, treated, not-treated and it was all bad once inside my mouth. It was like drinking aluminum from a tap. I stuck with the milk, juices and sports drinks until my neighbours offered me a taste of their well water. It was much better than anything else I'd tried. They were sweet enough to keep sending jugs of "the good stuff" for me.

At this stage, there were fewer time-out spells on the couch during the day. With Sharon's help I managed to get Skype downloaded and running on my laptop, an undertaking I would not have attempted the week previous. I was feeling so good I could almost say I was ready to do it all again. Give me another round. But then I realized there were still lingering symptoms. I was like an engine running on three of four cylinders. Not all there but running. Eleven days to Round Two. "Burp . . . honey . . . where are the antacids?"

Two weeks to the day after receiving the first round of chemo I absent-mindedly tugged and my hair came out in a clump. I just stared at it. I am talking about a wad of 40 long strands at one yank. Or more. I checked the other side of my head. Yank. Whoa. Fifty or more that time as well.

As usual, I knew but never truly believed it was going to happen.

Why was that? It's because I always think of myself as lucky. I figured I would be among that rare one percent who only suffered hair thinning. Not until I held the clumps in my hand did I realize I was in the larger group.

It was like ironing. Mom used to spend hours every day ironing basket loads of clothes. They would hang in her closet, sometimes for months, before being worn again. That meant she usually had to touch them up with an iron before wearing them. Eventually all clothes drift to the back of the closet, hidden behind the new items. Mom would stuff all the old, ironed clothes into plastic bags and send them to the Goodwill; all that ironing gone to waste.

The redundancy of it nearly drove me batty. I rarely iron anything, certainly not days in advance of wearing it. So why worry about chemo side effects beforehand? They might not come to pass. Yet here it was, in my hand. My hair.

Although a bit of a shocker for everyone, it made for a great practical joke. "Get a load of this," I told anyone I ran into. Then I tugged at a spot and out came a wad. Yep, big eyes right away; made me laugh every time.

My morning shower was a disaster. I couldn't get the hair off my wet hands and was that a guinea pig trying to go down the drain? I dressed and shuffled off to see my stylist Carolyn again. We decided to forgo razoring and clip it shorter, hoping enough stayed intact for the annual Ducks Unlimited dinner and auction on Saturday. My husband was the treasurer and sat at the door all night to either record what you'd bought or take your donations. I spent the night entering draws and shopping, a yearly highlight.

"If you notice any bald patches between now and then, we'll deal with it," Carolyn assured me. *With what? A felt-tipped marker?* I wondered.

But, for the time being, I still had my own hair! Extremely short but . . . tug-tug . . . it was still . . . oops! Got to quit that if I want any left for Saturday. Of course we did have two wigs on standby. Another bonus from the Smithers cancer unit. There were baskets of multicoloured styles from which to choose. I selected a blonde shag with a ring of brunette locks around the base. Exotic, I figured. Something to spice up my life.

There is a wig shop in Prince George where a wonderful woman spent an hour helping me decode what shade and shape best suited my face. She also introduced me to a skullcap, a thin nylon or cotton liner to fit beneath the wig. It provided instant relief from itching and kept the fake locks in place. She showed me how to line up the wig's side tabs with my ears to ensure it was on straight.

On November 18 it was minus 20 with five inches of fresh snow on the ground. The sun glittered against the crystal blue sky. I had to shade my eyes but there was a wide grin on my face. I couldn't re-call feeling that alive, that charged with energy, in years. Everything smelled better, tasted better (except for raspberries and water), and *was* better.

I did the circuit training class that morning and nudged the treadmill speed up to eight a few times. My feet were on fire, they moved so fast. Everyone was very obliging to the supercharged cancer girl and moved aside as I ran to each weight station, my stubby hair poking out at every angle. I felt like roaring! I was alive and strong and healthy . . . well, sort of. As I said to my husband, "Keep anyone in a dark hole long enough . . ." It was like I finally caught a break. I was able to (almost) feel like me again. I had returned; scarred, lighter, with less hair and breast tissue but I was up and running, swimming, walking, eating. The mouth sores were almost gone and I could actually feel the waning of the chemo's toxicity. Round One was almost over.

I was determined to use this energy in preparation for the next chemo session due in six days. More baking, bed changing, cleaning and smelling the roses. Heck, jumping over the roses and back again! Backflips, somersaults, tumbling, tumbling, tumbling.

It was finally a good day.

9

The First Sign of Trouble

Between my short hairdo and eye-popping two-inch false eye-lashes, I had felt like the belle of the ball at the Ducks Unlimited auction and dinner. I figured my not winning anything, despite a hundred draws among 90 people, meant all my luck had gone into catching my cancer early. Actually, I'd been lucky to have any hair left at all. The itchiness had been telling me for days that my hair was dead at the roots. What was left was illusional plumage held in place by the thinnest layer of magnetism to my body. Balls of hair had to be vacuumed off my pillow the next morning. At first the hair came out in my brush, heavier than normal. By day two, a soft tug resulted in fistfuls of long strands coming out. So I did not pull or tug at it, merely patted conditioner into it while showering then blotting it. Finger comb, no blow-drying. Thankfully, that helped it last another 10 days for the banquet.

My friend Kerri was wearing a scarf a few weeks into her chemo and I recall laughing at her. You can't have lost it already, I said, so she showed me the moonscape of her head. A definite clear-cut! It was shocking to see her baldness. I wasn't prepared for it and it showed.

I felt bad and told her so. I thanked Kerri for sharing her experi-ence. I knew that having some of my real hair at the banquet would give my friends and acquaintances time to adjust to the fact I was battling cancer, that the next time they saw me I'd be bald or wearing a head wrap or wig.

My after-banquet morning shower produced a towel so thickly coated in strands I imagined a dog had rolled on it and his coat had come off. And nothing prepares you for seeing islands of skin poking through your ocean of hair. It was so unnatural. Barry found some shears and, with my head in the garbage can, we laughed and cried and shaved the remaining hairs off. I watched the locks pile up. They were golden with black ends. I saved some but still don't know why. Then I looked in the mirror again. I didn't recognize myself. I looked like a man. I was *all* face with black peach fuzz dotting the surface of my scalp like patches of grit clinging to a glacier.

Stop it! Quit talking like that!

Baldness, I reminded myself, was my badge of honour. A statement of the difficulties I had been through and continued to face. It was an elite pass into a world of amazing people who faced their mortality square on. Our lives were changing. Like butterflies-to-be, we were metamorphosing into something beyond the busy, self- and time-absorbed people we had been. We had to prepare for the worst as there was no denying any of us only had so long to be here. When you have cancer, that fact stares you in the face. You re-evaluate your life, question your goals and prepare for the day you can leave without regret. This makes you patient about things. Changing the colour of the sofa pillows to better match the walls drops on the priority list.

Life had slowed down to a pace I could handle. I liked this speed much better. The day's entire agenda was going to be learning to look in the mirror and see past the physical. What I wanted to see was the brave person I knew was in there. When I succeeded at that, I might just crawl back into bed for a nap. At least I wouldn't need to vacuum my pillow afterwards.

The second chemo session on December 2 went by without so

much drama. Barry's offer to accompany me was accepted with a kiss and we were joined by two friends who helped the time pass quickly. A footbath of ice water was prepared at my insistence, still worried as I was about losing my toenails.

The cycle repeated itself with the post-chemo, full-on energy, thanks to the steroids, followed by a precipitous drop into the symptom basement. This time it was easier because I knew what to do, which foods to avoid, which ones helped. I knew to always keep a Popsicle or gum within arm's reach. My mouth was forever dry so I was drinking Gatorade and juices, which seemed to work for everything but my waistline. I tried not to think about that. Determined to keep some of my old self, I continued sluggishly with the aqua fitness, jogging and circuit training. I talked incessantly so that my mind wouldn't know what I was putting my body through. It wasn't hard to fool myself. I had a bad case of what they called "chemo brain": thinking and memory problems experienced by many cancer survivors. Things were slow to enter and quick to exit. I felt aware and cognizant, then couldn't remember one thing I had said or done mere minutes ago. People started looking at me funny after a conversation. I didn't make much sense. I had the IQ and attention span of a gumdrop. In short, I was not running on all cylinders for at least a year. I identified with every blonde joke ever told. Not that I could remember any.

On a more positive note, my dear friend Jane was due to arrive and I got weepy at the thought. A lot of things were making me weep — thoughts about the kids coming home for the holidays, the new water cooler in the kitchen and the Christmas television reruns. By the time Frosty the Snowman melted I was sobbing.

Jane's arrival gave me a burst of fake energy. Instead of relaxing as I was supposed to, we decorated the house, wrapped presents, baked, made desserts and visited way past my bedtime. I was like a cyclone in the morning, a slight breeze by noon and still air by mid-afternoon. That's when Jane would force me to lie down before rubbing my feet with cream while we listened to a soothing Gregorian chant CD. It was church music from the early Middle Ages, spiritual and soothing. I often fell into a peaceful sleep.

Other than tiredness, the cold bald head and the internal issues for which I took pills, things were manageable. Morale wavered at times. I felt so beaten up, so dragged through the mud by my ankles. I wondered how slow I'd be by the fourth chemo session. Ever watched a turtle move? The thought made me smile. Yet turtles don't sink, they swim. Good analogy!

My radiation appointment was January 15th in Kelowna so we had to start making plans. We would be there for at least six weeks, possibly eight. We wouldn't know until the consult, also on the 15th. I was resigned to waiting once again. And I did that so well.

December 8 was the first and hopefully last birthday where I had to be careful that my candles didn't set my synthetic hair on fire. I also had to watch the dishwasher on steam cycle and had been warned not to pull a turkey or any baked things from a hot oven. The bangs on my wig would shrivel irreparably, making me look like one of my sister's old Barbie dolls after our brother took a match to it. I didn't want my hair's fate to be the same as Barbie's when we couldn't get rid of the burnt glue smell. I'd be down to wearing do-rags on my head for the rest of the process.

The fake hair was worn mainly for show. At home, alone, I wore a soft, under-helmet beanie from a ski shop or wrapped my pate in one of the many colourful scarves given to me by friends. My neighbors probably thought I'd changed religions.

At five one morning, I'd been awake for a few hours just lying in bed doing my usual "diagnostic tests." Mentally, I sorted through my body parts, seeing how they felt. There was an ache in both knees, a slight fever I needed to check with the thermometer and the metallic taste was waning. The headaches of the past four days had subsided but a burn in my chest had me wondering if I was coming down with something. I hadn't been the best of patients during my low-immunity week. Instead of avoiding people, I invited a bunch of women over for a makeup party.

One sunny morning after the party Jane and I tried to run half of our old jogging route. I had to stop three times to catch my breath. I couldn't seem to get enough air in. A deep breath made me cough. Nothing hurt, I simply couldn't breathe enough.

"SLOW DOWN," they said (Barry, Jane, Sandi, Dr. Z, etc., etc., ad infinitum).

"I'm off to the ski hill," I said. It was a fresh powder weekend. Or we had company. Or there was a birthday party for a friend. There was always something going on. I wanted so bad to keep things as normal as possible. Cancer? What cancer? Yes, I am my own worst enemy.

Our ski cabin has a cozy couch and five beds with plush blankets and pillows if I need them. And they're far enough from the fireplace I wouldn't need to worry about my wig shriveling into gnarled plastic. "Come on, let's go!"

The wheezing got worse.

My birthday card from Jane had a picture of a mouse about to attempt stealing the cheese from a loaded mouse trap. It was wearing a miniature helmet.

What was life without some optimism?

I was officially 51 but I cried like I was 10 as Jane boarded the plane. I waved until my arm hurt and the plane was long out of sight.

Buck up, I thought. Through her positivity, spirituality and peacefulness Jane had supplied me with my own helmet, now strapped tightly to my bald head. Time to go get the cheese and survive this ordeal.

The days passed slowly, so each card or letter I found waiting for me at the end of a 20-minute walk to the post box lifted my soul. Some days I marched to that box and on others I dragged a rusted,

100-pound ache behind me, but I got there. It was every friend that came over to see how I was doing, staying for a nice, distracting talk over a steaming cup of tea, most likely dropping off flowers, a casserole, soup, muffins, a bag of fruit. It was my sister's flood of gifts to help improve my circumstance, like sending Homer to help me through the scary things. There were constant phone calls from all over the world, the best being from Dad to say he loved me. These were busy people with busy lives taking a moment to let me know they cared. It was overwhelming and it lifted me up and away from myself again and again. I was enveloped by love during what was starting to feel like a never-ending road. Although my faith in recovery wavered like a little kid at the edge of the high diving board, none of my friends ever did. My life was in their hands and they never let me down. They propped me up and I can never thank them enough. You can bet I'll be there for them if they ever need the favour returned.

My chemo sessions were scheduled 21 days apart. On day 19 I had blood tests done and on day 20 I was in to see Dr. Z regarding the results and to discuss the next treatment. We were surprised that the counts were all great because the shortness of breath I had been experiencing for over a week was worse. Walking from downstairs to the upper level of the house flattened me.

Then we went to the ski hill. The first few runs of the day were okay but I was shaky and breathless riding the T-bar lift back up. By afternoon I had to stop four times on the journey down. I never had to do that. I'm usually a T-to-B (top to bottom) girl but now I sounded like a chain saw skiing down Chapman's Challenge. Who was that old lady with the bronchitis?

I told myself the snow was thick and tougher to push through. Barry figured it meant my red blood cell count was down, which would be normal while having chemotherapy. Red blood cells carry oxygen to every cell in your body. It sounded reasonable but my blood work said everything was fine. "Your stats are healthy . . . something must be terribly wrong."

So, before continuing with the next chemo session, Dr. Z had to rule out possibilities like pulmonary embolism. A pulmonary embolism occurs when a blood clot breaks from its initial location and travels into the lungs. Once there, serious complications quickly arise. If that was happening, I was in real danger.

Phone calls to Terrace were made within minutes. If I could be there by 2 p.m. the hospital could squeeze in an emergency CT scan. Could I make it alone through a building snow storm?

What? Could I jump the next hurdle standing between me and getting this ordeal over with? Is that what you're asking? Stand back, everyone. Someone might get hurt (like me) but I'm going to try it anyway. Thank goodness I hadn't eaten any lunch as you had to fast for four hours prior to the test. My cup of herbal tea on the drive to Smithers didn't count. I was good to go.

All I had was two and a half hours to get to a place that normally took two on a clear, quiet day. With white knuckles on the steering wheel I guided our tank-like Suburban down the snow-covered highway. I could barely see where the road ended and the shoulder began. Traffic had slowed to a crawl but I couldn't crawl with them. I was on a timer that might change my life. If there was something wrong it would have to be dealt with immediately. Would they have to keep me in the Terrace hospital for a while? I hadn't thought of that. I hadn't brought anything.

But that was the least of what troubled me. If the chemo had to be delayed, that would mess with the schedule I had figured out for Christmas. The kids were coming and I didn't want them to see me going through the worst of the post-treatment woes. It would ruin Christmas and upset them. Maybe Christmas would have to be cancelled. That thought resulted in almond-sized tears which blurred my vision.

The driving went from scary to "get the heck off the road." I swayed and fishtailed my way past multiple logging trucks and transports kicking up blinding clouds of snow. My stomach whined and moaned. It was empty and knotted. My nerves were shredded. I was passing vehicles in the ditch, skid marks still visible across the highway and through the snow banks.

What was I doing?

Stop thinking and drive!

I arrived in Terrace wigless and pale with eight minutes to spare. I had endured 10 hot flashes on the journey. That's one every 15 minutes. Sitting in the hospital parking lot after all that seemed so anticlimactic. Where was the finish line ribbon, the floral wreaths, the congratulations? Smarter questions might have been "How many days had been subtracted from my life due to the stress of that trip? And when would the shaking stop?"

Terrace, being much closer to the coast than Houston, was a massive slush puddle. Think of a frozen margarita stained brown with road dirt. I had a soaker in my ankle-high leather boot within minutes of trying to walk from the tank to hospital admitting.

I checked in and was herded straight to the testing area where I was gowned, stretchered, IV'd and placed under the CT beams. Like the MRI scanner, the CT machine is a big round donut. I was in the hole. Dye was injected through my IV so fast I experienced a warm flushing sensation. I felt like I had to pee and it got so warm between my legs I worried maybe I had.

Then the tests were finished. The good news was my underwear was dry and even better, no embolism. Okay, time to take stock again. It was three o'clock and the storm outside was still raging. I was exhausted, starving and it was starting to get dark. In less than an hour it would be pitch black. By December 21st, the shortest day of the year, we get only five hours of sunlight a day.

I called my friend Terry, who invited me to stay the night. But first we'd have dinner at my favourite restaurant. With that arranged,

I headed downtown to buy a toothbrush, clean underwear and dry footwear. It wouldn't do to catch pneumonia at this stage of the game. Within the hour my feet were encased in dry, tall, shiny, black boots. They were my size, 50 percent off and they lifted my spirits. Watch out everyone. Mrs. Claus is coming through. Ho, ho, ho.

I enjoyed a much-needed night of girl talk with Terry before heading home in the morning on clearer, ploughed roads. It was a leisurely, one-hot-flash trip.

While I'd been gone, Dr. Z had contacted the oncologist in Kelowna who wanted a few more tests, like an echocardiogram for my heart and something else more complicated that required a radiologist to be present. More waiting. And no chemo until we get this resolved. I figured (ha!) the fatigue and shortness of breath maybe resulted from a touch of the flu but my caregivers were being careful. It did occur to me that maybe they would postpone the chemo until after Christmas. The kids could have the real me with some pink in my cheeks. Of course, that would also mean I'd be cooking Christmas dinner and not just barking out orders? Hmmm.

I told myself it was out of my hands. Things happened for a reason and I truly believe that. Take those shiny new boots. How could that possibly be a fluke? If they had been full price I would not have been able to justify buying them. I wouldn't have bought them at 20 or 30 or even 40 percent off . . . but 50 percent? That was my song. I was needy and karma provided. I could never find boots that fit and were on sale. And I mean never!

The world worked in mysterious ways.

"You're such a loveable flake," my sister told me on the inside of an appropriate card that said "What shoes go with this stress?"

10

Hair Loss 101

The evening before my scheduled chemo date I took the anti-nauseate just in case I was declared healthy by 9:30 in the morning and we could proceed like none of the wheezing and shortness of breath ever happened. I know . . . it was another pie-in-the-sky bit of thinking, totally unbacked by anyone but me, but if you couldn't believe in a few miracles now and again . . . I mean, hey, it was Christmas! It's not like I was asking for two front teeth.

And, while lying in bed awake at 3 a.m., I started thinking baldness deserved its own segment in this book. I needed to tell everyone about *all* the baldness because the burning question my friends wanted to ask was not "How does chemo feel?" — it was "Exactly what hair do you lose while on chemotherapy?"

Okay. Chemo Baldness 101. Two weeks after administration of the first doses of docetaxel and cyclophosphamide the hair on my head could be tugged out in clumps and needed to be shaved off. Either that or ignore the trail of hairy dust bunnies following me. The hair under my arms and on my legs disappeared and, yes, the hair that declares I'm about as naturally blonde as burnt toast had thinned to almost non-existence. Would it grow back grey like the hair on my head might? Egad! As if there wasn't already enough mental and physical scarring to deal with. Grey pubic hair. Can you dye that?

Last and by far the *least* burning question from everyone was about the facial hair which grew along the jaw line. My husband chose to point this out in front of company one night. The instinctive kick he got on his shin looked harsher than it was. But it took the attention away from my embarrassment. Maybe this was something I should attempt to deal with. I had been hoping it would just fall out like everything else. Barry didn't seem to think I might be sensitive about something he faced daily. What? What's the big deal about a beard?

Waxing was not the answer for me. I had a bad experience which comes out later in the book . . . and the resounding holler could be heard for miles. I tried the depilatory cream but it felt like it was eating my skin. Razoring was out of the question. But I did succumb to the no!no! hair removal system as seen on the late night shopping channel. It's a controversial item that works for some. I love it for facial hair.

My eyebrows and lashes were the last to go and, strangely, the first things to grow back. I didn't dare give them the tug test. Can you imagine missing half an eye of lash? I have never figured out how to apply false lashes but I did glue my eyes shut once.

It's strange that most of my body hair just disappeared while spots of fuzz on my head survived. Little Velcro-like tufts that attached me to my pillowcase, picked at my silk scarves and anchored my wig. I had a permanent five o'clock shadow atop my skull as well as black, pokey patches on the sideburn areas that were sometimes visible. That's why I had to shave my head every other day, which made me feel like a phony.

"Look, she's not bald. She's shaving her head voluntarily."

I was feeling shameful about the parts of my head that were not barren. How twisted is that? Was it because I didn't fit into what I assumed a chemo patient went through? Leave it to me to lose my hair the wrong way. Could I do nothing right?

I did warn the kids I didn't look quite the same. Yes, they'd heard from friends here in town that I looked fine, upbeat, made-up, walking with my chin held high. But, I told them, they would be privy to the other person whose wig ended up trampled on the floor mat of the car after the itchiness wore me down or when a hot flash made it impossible to leave on. They would see me so tired I slumped like discarded tissue, weariness pulling my unmasked facial features into all-new lows. Never mind a facelift. I needed a tractor pull. I had aged to Betty White status. In fact, I think Betty looked younger.

I called it my Chemo Countenance. My face, whether I liked it or not, reflected many things — the strain of the treatments, the surgeries, the guilt of eating too much chocolate, the worry that a family member or friend might end up on this road. Yet I had to believe one could see the hope that was there, the future with weddings and grandkids and a life without trauma and sickness. I hoped my kids would remember my usual vibrant smiling face. When I thought about it, my life was pretty wonderful, facial hair or no hair at all.

I spent the morning of the day I was supposed to have Chemo Number Three getting another blood test and lining up an echocardiogram when a radiologist could be present. We were trying to rule out any heart damage possibly caused by the previous doses of chemo or, more likely, by my unwillingness to slow down while on the treatments. I was so bad for myself. Why did I have to push myself when my body was already fighting the battle of a lifetime?

I was still wheezing, unable to get enough air when exerting myself even the tiniest bit. I felt like this years ago when we were in Cuzco, Peru, where the air is so thin. Trying to run more than 15 feet left me gasping for air in the street. I never fully acclimatized to Cuzco even though I drank the recommended 10 cups of coca tea a day. I did, however, become very mellow and calm for the first time in my life. Too bad coca tea is illegal in Canada.

Normally one has to travel to Prince George or Terrace for the echocardiogram, but the stars had once again aligned and a radiologist would be coming to Smithers on Friday. He was overbooked due to the Christmas holidays but agreed to come in early and do this. Again, I silently thanked Mom, my own personal Santa Claus who was somehow managing to steer good luck and fortune my way, before getting out the recipe books and baking some white chocolate, cranberry muffins. Put together with fresh oranges and bananas, it made a nice basket for the doctor and staff to share. It was "Thanks!" and a gesture aimed at paving the way for the next patient in need of something above and beyond the call of someone's duty.

I was given a steroid inhaler to see if it eased some of the problem. My husband put on his pharmacist cap to show me more than once how to push the button and inhale the mist deeply into my lungs. It was easier when I stopped talking but, besides making me a bit light-headed, it didn't seem to have any effect on my wheezing.

I hoped I would be declared fit enough to get back to the chemo soon. But any chemo now meant the kids would see me during the worst days. I would be at my all-time lowest on Christmas Day. Another consideration was that too much time between chemo treatments lessened effectiveness. Better to check all the vitals, make sure I could take another round, then full steam ahead.

For the most part my life followed its normal patterns. I just couldn't run for the phone or work out. My big exercise for the day was lifting a fork to my mouth . . . in a house loaded with chocolaty, gooey Christmas baking. I was not supposed to be eating any sugar but at least I made everything with 70 percent dark chocolate. That meant the new blobs of fat on my backside would be healthier than usual.

By December 18 my wonderful girlfriend Jane had come and gone, leaving a festive glow throughout our home. The decorated Christmas tree shimmered above dozens of carefully wrapped presents, many sporting flashy bows or ribbons. As tradition went at our house, we each got to open one present on December 24th, but I couldn't wait that long.

I chose the massive square box from my in-laws containing a mini-trampoline. The pressure under my arm had been building since the swimming stopped. It was called lymph node backup and it needed to be drained. Ten minutes of light bouncing up and down on a trampoline would decompress the area and, if I was lucky, take away my cares and burn some chocolate calories.

Okay, not all my cares. I was still frustrated by the imminent chemo situation. How bad was it going to mess up our Christmas? No one wanted to see their mother when she was thinking about throwing herself in front of a train. Maybe if I could convince the cancer unit to wait and give me the chemo on December 24th, nine days late, I would still feel like taking part in our annual seafood dinner that night, opening gifts in the morning and eating Christmas dinner. I usually got very sick, tired and suffered the worst on days three to five. That would be December 26 to 28. The wheels never stopped turning. I had to make this work. Think. Think!

We had been wearing our portable phones like necklaces, waiting for news from the Kelowna oncologist. I was stressed to the point of cold sores on my upper lip, a big zit on my nose and sighing heavily every few minutes. The kids were not the only problem a late chemo date might incur. I had a radiation appointment in Kelowna for January 19th and changing the chemo date might change that date, which meant having to hassle a lot of people to change plans concerning our travel and accommodation. This became a front-line fret. I became irritable about everything, swinging at life like it was a big nasty piñata.

Then, on December 23rd, the call came and it was the greatest gift I ever received. It didn't come with wrapping or a bow, but it was a Christmas gift unlike any other. The oncologist decided I'd had enough. It had been debatable how much chemo I needed in the first place with such a micro metastasis. They had wreaked enough damage on my body, Dr. KJ said, and anything further could be unnecessarily detrimental. Get out of jail free. Proceed directly to radiation in January. Have a nice Christmas!

After I hung up the phone I sat down and stared into space. What did that even mean? How could they say I needed a certain amount of chemo, then say I didn't? That I'd had enough? Did they know what they were doing? Shouldn't I be scared that they wouldn't give me what they'd convinced me was necessary?

I went upstairs and gave the news to Barry. He crossed the kitchen with a half empty glass of rum and Coke in his hand. He wrapped his arms around me and started to cry. My husband does not cry very often and, regrettably, I reacted poorly. A feeling of intense anger crept up. He was supposed to be a rock. How could he fall apart when this was far from over? It must be the alcohol. I pushed him away from me and stalked out of the room. Yes, I felt bad, horrible even. I was an emotional wreck and, as usual, wouldn't let Barry in. I fell asleep worrying maybe the wrong decision had been made about the chemo. It was the answer to my prayers for a wonderful Christmas with the kids, but was it going to cost me my life? How could we know for certain this was the right thing to do?

I was very scared for the next two days. It took reassurance from Sandi and the cancer unit nurses that I had been given more chemo than others for the same amount of cancer. I *should* be okay. I would be on one and perhaps two anti-cancer drugs as soon as the radiation was completed. I needed to relax a bit because I was in good hands. Here I was feeding the bad cells with stress again. I might as well have crammed a box of chocolate bars down my throat, washing them along with an entire bottle of Merlot. It was me I should be afraid of, not the cancer.

At first it was hard to loosen up because I didn't trust anything anymore. The world felt like it was made of rice paper and would vanish. But slowly the gift the oncologist had given us began to outweigh any fear. Surprise and concern were replaced by excitement and energy. I did a complete 360. I never felt so blessed, so spoiled in my entire life. Who else in the world got a pass on chemo at Christmas? This was better than any wish I could have imagined.

There would be no IV of chemical waste a day or two before Christmas. No feeling like I'd been run down by Santa and all 12 reindeer. No mouth sores, numbness or metallic turkey taste. No heartburn and aches and night sweats and terrors. I was done with the chemo stage of the horror story and could concentrate on my family, on Christmas and growing some hair. I would take a break from being sick.

My holiday began with a meek apology to my husband who, uncharacteristically, held his tongue, and we made up as best we could. Then another day flew by and my daughter, my son, and his gal Debra arrived. I was overjoyed and shocked. Lorne had shaved his head and Karly had her long locks lobbed off. Why would they do that to themselves? They admitted it had not been for a fundraiser. It had been for me. I was dumbfounded. Who the heck wanted to look like this? Then I heard my nephew Zach had done the same thing. I relished the thought that they wanted to support me, but as an afterthought there are better ways. Be interested in who I am and what I want, like helping to prevent more people from getting cancer. Listen to what I have to say and spread the word. Clean up your own life in honour of me. Better yet, do it for yourself. That would be an extra-special gift for anyone dealing with cancer!

Still, hairy or not, that Christmas was one of the best ever and I would not have changed a thing. We put on warm toques and laughed and ate and went skiing on our mountain. It was just what this weary soul needed. My strength and vitality grew every day. I was never as aware of the good things in my life. My determination to stick around for years to come to be with my children and their families renewed itself. I wanted to be there for them for as long as I could. For years longer than my mom had made it. Amazing what the power of love, mixed with some good news for a change, could do.

And then it was the New Year and I was into another anxiety-ridden holding pattern, waiting this time for a consult with the radiation oncologist in Kelowna. We were trying to get the date moved up because chemo had ended six weeks early and I was not on any anti-cancer drug regime yet. If the chemo did miss anything it could be growing. Every sugared bite of Christmas junk or slurp of heavily egg-nogged chai tea made me worry (after it had passed my lips, of course) I had fanned a cancerous spark into flame. I had done what I'd done and enjoyed Christmas and New Year's to the max. Now I was going to pay for it. The worry of a recurrence hung over my head and zapped my butt with a thunderbolt of guilt with every memory of a sinful treat. It's good I can take a lot of pain.

While in this holding pattern I decided to transform from recovering surgery-chemo patient back to a writer-exercise fanatic who counted calories. My resolution was to spend less time trying to numb myself with games, books and movies and use that energy in a constructive way. I had allotted enough to this cancer thing. It was time to reclaim my life, albeit with occasional timeouts for medical appointments and travel. The difference during what I called Phase Three (surgery and chemo being the first two phases) of this entire health debacle would be the mindset. Everything in my life did not have to be about cancer.

It was time to hang the Do Not Disturb sign on my office door again. Not because I was having a nap, but because I was back to writing. Okay, maybe a bit of both in the beginning.

Having all this energy back (and hair, although it was merely salt & pepper peach fuzz) lifted my spirits to the moon. We spent the first weekend in January ripping up the fresh powder on our local Hudson Bay Mountain. I was not quite back to doing top-to-bottoms but I was out there in the pine-scented cool surrounded by friends and good, clean fun. The never-ending hot flashes were a breeze when I was on a chairlift at minus 10. I just ripped off my hat.

But that's not the best of what happened on the ski hill. My dentist, the hot, young Dr. Yummy, was skiing on the mountain that weekend. I'd seen him there before but didn't usually get the chance to talk to him. He asked if he could ride up with me on the T-bar. I agreed with a nod of my head because, as usual, this man took my breath away. Thank goodness I had my wig and hat on. It didn't hide the deformities I felt inside, but it helped hide the ugliness on the outside.

We chatted about the weather and skiing before he asked how I was, how I *really* was. He knew about the cancer. I told him that I thought my days of tabletop dancing were over. It was a joke I'd used when around close friends. The words fell out of my mouth before I could stop them.

He grinned and told me, "You don't need to have a nice body or hair to be beautiful, because you *are* beautiful."

It was amazing I didn't fall right off the lift.

I looked away and then whispered, "What can I say to that? But thank you."

"I have to be careful here because you are my patient," he reminded me, letting me know he wasn't flirting, "but you are. You're beautiful."

"Thanks," I mumbled once more. I mean really, what *could* you say? No one had ever said this to me out of the blue before, like it was a conversational topic, especially not when I'd needed to hear it more than ever in my life. His timing was epic. Had he known that? The crinkled skin around his eyes and his wide grin said possibly he did.

Please don't get my good dentist wrong. He had a girlfriend, maybe even "the one." He was just trying to help me see beyond the externalities. And it worked. It worked because whatever my flaws, someone out there thought I was beautiful. It made me feel like I didn't have to cover up, to hide myself, to shrink away. And this handsome young man had taken the time to make sure I was aware of it. Dr. Y restored my dignity and there are moments when I feel he also saved my sanity, which can be close to the same thing for some of us.

I have replayed that scene at least 1,000 times. Over the next year I would hear those words each and every time I looked in the mirror and saw the freakish, twisted boob, the hairless, old woman who resembled a greying turtle. Like the pass from chemo, it was a gift like none other. I again gave my mother credit. She had put Dr. Y into my life for a reason and there it was.

I finally received the call from Kelowna saying my radiation appointment was not going to change. It would be January 19th for the consult and the pretests. However, my first treatment would be five days sooner . . . "Fry-day," January 28.

That left nine days to fritter away in Kelowna. Maybe we would get in some skiing and do a little shopping. The modest inheritance from my mother could be appropriately spent at a ski shop. After only four years my current skis had delaminated across the tops. They were unsafe and looked like something I had picked up at a yard sale. They had to go. Mom had been a skier right to the end, strapping on the boards even after her cancer diagnosis. I couldn't think of a better way to spend her money. Thanks again, Mom.

11

Saving My Dignity

It was minus 10 when we arrived in the Okanagan and there was fresh snow on the ground. Road conditions had been good and our new Suburban performed well. It had arrived in Houston the previous week, replacing the one I totaled earlier. Seven months after Mom died I had been going east on Highway 16 when a westbound van turned left in front of me. My old Suburban went from 90 kilometres per hour to zero in a split second. When I felt it was safe to open my eyes, I saw the airbag from my steering wheel smoking and shrinking away from me.

It was 5:45 in the morning. I had been headed to the gym to work out with Sandi.

The police said I was lucky I had been driving a heavy-duty SUV and had sustained "only" a bad case of whiplash. I didn't put it down to luck. It was Mom's first attempt at a miracle and I silently gave credit to where I thought it was due. Eventually there was a cash settlement as a result of the accident, enough to pay for the luxury of physio and massage therapy for the whiplash and the partial mastectomy area for many years to come.

As I said, the replacement Suburban came right before we left for the Cancer Centre of the Southern Interior (CCSI) in Kelowna.

The smell of new leather got me high and the heated seats and command start filled me with insane joy.

My uncle and his wife were away on holidays and graciously lent us their home, a 15-minute jog from the CCSI. I made a run there and back, checking out where to park and what route we should drive. It was my first jog since my lungs turned wheezy a month ago and it felt inspiring to be back at it. I went slow and found I wasn't breathing hard at all; it was only when I tried to race or speed up that I got winded.

It was strange at first, being in a relative's house without the relatives, but we soon unpacked and settled in. We dragged in two coolers of salmon and halibut, caught by Barry in the summer, and some of the moose meat and grouse he had hunted in the fall. One plastic tub held my favourite healthy recipe books, packages of brown rice pasta and spices. It was great to be able to cook what I wanted how I wanted instead of relying on restaurants. I was in complete control of my diet (which doesn't mean I was always in good hands).

The upcoming meeting with medical oncologist Dr. KJ and radiation oncologist Dr. R had been a long time coming. I felt like a battle-weary soldier heading to the command post to get my next orders. They were my generals leading the charge against the cancer cooties. That made them VIPs in my life. Like rock stars. OMG. What was I going to wear?

Just *kidding*!

I was nervous because I was about to find out the answers to two very important questions. First, whether or not my underarm had to be radiated as well as my breast area, possibly heading me toward an increased risk of lymphedema, the swelling that can become permanent. I had lost faith in my cancer luck (still not convinced that the Christmas pass on chemo had been for the best) and had steeled myself for anything. "They will probably miss my breast and zap my heart," I quipped, worrying now that I'd said it

I'd jinxed myself. "I'd be on fire for you, baby," I told my husband, unsuccessfully trying to make light of my anxiety.

The other answer I was about to receive concerned my length of stay in the Okanagan. Barry did relief work as a pharmacist and could take off as much time as he needed and my writing went where I went. But our home would be missing us before long and we would be missing our friends, our food, our mail, our routine.

I dressed in easily-removed layers in case my nerves brought on multiple hot flashes and threw a battery-operated hand fan into my purse.

Live piano music floats around the foyer of the Kelowna cancer clinic every day at noon, which was when we arrived. I walked toward the receptionist, who instructed us to go down the hall and turn left. "In the fishbowl waiting area," she said, smiling at my puzzled expression. "You can't miss it."

She was right. You couldn't miss the giant fish tank filled with a rainbow of fish. I took a seat and was given a questionnaire by a very efficient nurse named Dave. A free coffee/tea cart circled by me for the third time . . . "Sure I can't whip you up a cuppa?" the silver-haired volunteer coaxed. I finally conceded and felt grateful as my jittery fingers wrapped around the steaming waxed container. Barry opted out.

Classy, I mused, checking out the clean design of the building and the way everything seemed to run so smoothly. It had to. The numbers through those doors every day were astounding and the saddest news was that the faces were ever changing. There was no age restriction with cancer. You only had to be alive to grow it. You only had to be dead to get away from it completely.

Dave, who worked for Dr. KJ, ushered me into an examination room and went over my questionnaire answers, noting where all four of our kids lived and asking about their health as well as Barry's.

Dave laughed at the answer to *Why are you here?* I had put "I'm lonely" and for *Sex?* "Often." I filled out the important parts properly: menses started at age 13, five operations to date and climbing.

It had only been two and a half months since we'd met via video conference at the Smithers hospital but Dr. KJ looked quite different. I hadn't realized she was pregnant and due in another few months. Just the concept of babies thrilled me at this stage of my life. We needed more babies to balance the world out. People died and right behind them someone was born. The Circle of Life. It made me want to smile. Instead, I had a massive hot flash and made quite the scene of wrestling out of three layers of coat, scarf and sweater.

Once I settled down, we were ready to start, Barry with a pen and paper ready to record everything. The doctor was pleased with the progress to date and said they would not be radiating my armpit area but would deliver 16 treatments directed at the right breast tissue. That was the short, three-week course, meaning our complete stay in Kelowna would only be for five weeks! My luck was holding after all.

My next meeting was with Dr. R, the radiation oncologist. She performed a brief physical examination, as she had never met me before, and then, in one long breath, delivered a tightened explanation of what would happen, could happen and hopefully never happen to me . . . a talk you could tell she had given hundreds of times.

When she was finished I was welcomed to ask questions, but she had covered them all. I got her approval for the extra vitamins the naturopath recommended — vitamin D, multi B and the multivitamin — but I was not to take extreme doses.

The only intimidating part was hearing that a small bit of lung would inevitably get in the way and be radiated. There was no helping that.

"As long as I can still ski," I told her. "And hike. And swim. And run."

"I get the picture," she said. "It shouldn't be a problem for any of that."

We wished each other a nice day and went our separate ways, her to an inner office and me back to the fishbowl waiting area.

Next was the CT scan that would help the technicians map out the exact area to be radiated. I stripped from the waist up and put on the hospital gowns: one for the back, one for the front. These gowns were now mine to take home and care for during the 16 treatments. I wouldn't have to get new ones each visit. I imagine the time required to wash the gowns that people have on for mere minutes would be astounding; it made sense to ask everyone to wash their own.

A team of two female techs had me remove the front gown and lie on a steel cot. They stretched my right arm above my head to rest on a separate steel holder. The cot was raised by hydraulics another three feet higher in the air. My chest was completely exposed. I got drawn on with ink before two mini blue dots were tattooed onto my skin, one between my breasts and one on the right side of my right breast. It didn't really hurt, not like when I got the maple leaf tattoos on my leg. The little blue dots ensured I would never be radiated in this area again and also served as markers, defining the exact same treatment area for each visit.

The techs were very sweet and the entire procedure took only 30 minutes. They explained what would happen when I came for treatment. It would take 10 minutes to line me up and 10 minutes to zap me. This was going to be the easiest part of the whole treatment ordeal! My hand passed over my fuzzy head. Maybe the worst *had* passed?

I now had nine days off and would return a week Friday to receive my first treatment. Treatments would resume Monday to Friday for the next three weeks and then I would be free to go home.

On a last note, we left the clinic and headed to a pub for lunch. The waitress asked if I had come from the cancer clinic and I said that I had. (Was the do-rag on my head her first clue, or was I starting to really look like one of those cancer patients in the movies?)

We received 10 percent off our meals as clinic patients were VIPs. The gesture made me feel special and I thanked them.

I ordered a soothing cup of peppermint tea to make up for the pinch of the tattoo and vowed to return to the Pheasant and Quail in the near future. The bar was hosting a Super Bowl party February 6 and this bald head was going to be there. There would be lots of door prizes, which would have meant nothing to me the week prior. But now, it appeared my luck had returned. Only three weeks of radiation! We would be home by February 20th! Maybe with a Super Bowl prize tucked beneath my good arm? One had to keep optimistic in life.

With more than a week to wait before my first radiation appointment, we decided to stay and play. I had returned to what I'd guess was 85 percent of my former self; a heat flashing, sore and skeptical "me" but myself all the same. Back to swimming and jogging on alternate days and ripping up the powdery slopes at the Big White Ski Resort with our daughter Lindsay who has lived in Kelowna for five years.

As luck would again have it, we ran into a ski promotion day on the mountain. Several ski gear companies were letting the public try out their products for free. I danced a pair of hot Lady Salomons through the trees. I rode them hard and came up smiling. Wow. Like having rockets attached to my feet. They seemed easier to steer around branches and moguls than my old skis and I had to admit this would be the year to give myself a break. I was sold on everything but the price. I decided to wait longer into the season and hope for a sale.

I hopped onto my old skis and hit the runs. The day was warming up exceptionally and before long sweat was trickling down my back. Hot flashes and three layers of gear on my head didn't help. There was a fleece hat on top, my wig beneath and a thick skullcap under that. All cinched into place with a pair of goggles. Something had to go.

I heard a gasp in the lineup behind me as I reached up and pulled off all three layers. Steam rose from my bald head. It felt delicious. I reapplied the skullcap and toque, cinching it on with my goggles again and was good to go. Lindsay hadn't noticed until we got off the lift and thought maybe I had left my hair hanging on a tree. No, I assured her, my hair piece was safe inside my coat, held there by my powder-skirt, which snaps snug against my waist. These skirts are to keep the fine powder from travelling up into your jacket. Right now it would keep my hair from slipping *out* of my jacket.

After skiing, Lindsay and Barry went for a beer while I hit the shops in search of a ski suit. It was my Christmas gift from Barry but I had yet to find it. I was enjoying the search and it was a very enthusiastic me that threw my jacket to the ground at the outdoor rack of discounted suits at the first ski shop I found in the village. I tried on a dozen of every size and shape. Finding nothing, I collected my coat and went inside to investigate further. The lime Descente at the far end of the shop caught my eye as did the Spyder waist-to-coat zippers which make the latest outfit back into a one-piece.

I was removing a jacket when a young Australian girl who worked at the store approached and asked, "Excuse me . . . er, are you missing something?" At first I thought she meant my purse, a regular occurrence for me, but then I remembered I hadn't brought a purse. Then I got it . . . "Is it brown?" I asked. We both smiled as she produced something akin to roadkill. It was mangled and sopping wet, having been trampled by others who had checked out the bargains at the outdoor rack. I hoped my lost wig wouldn't be her favourite story from Canada.

I made my way to the bar to meet the others and, as I told them the story, I pulled out the wig and slipped it on. That drew a few eye-popping stares from other patrons at nearby tables.

You would think with the number of bald chemo patients on the rise, especially in a cancer clinic town like Kelowna, people might start getting used to the fact that not every full head of hair out there is what it seems. A kid can spot a wig in a second and will howl if you look at them sideways. What is it that unnerves people? There are multiple fake body parts available. Why should synthetic hair be uncool while silicone fingernails and butt implants are not? Is one phonier than the other?

I say whip those wigs off in front of the unsuspecting and get them used to it; like taking off a Band-Aid slowly or in one shot. Get over it, everyone.

Wigs can be a good thing, especially when you're hot flashing. How many menopausers can tear off their hair to cool down? Don't like your hair colour? Put on a different shade. Want long hair today? Maybe some dreadlocks for the first time in your life? Have at it.

Some of the wigs available can really change a person's look, like with Kerri, the friend with the clear-cut scalp. After losing her hair, she traded her look of curly long brown hair for a sporty straight blonde style and got *Wow*s everywhere she went.

The weather forecast said snow, snow and more snow so we decided to go to Revelstoke, a famous ski area three hours east in B.C.'s Kootenay Mountains. Still in holiday mode, we found a sweet three-day "stay and ski" deal online through the Sandman Inn. We booked a kitchenette so we could make our oatmeal, yogurt, seeds and blueberry breakfasts. Lunches would be at the restaurant on the slopes and dinners at one of the many great restaurants we remembered from all our previous adventures in the area. It had been four years since we'd skied Mount Mackenzie. Now called the Revelstoke Ski Resort, there were lifts to areas previously accessible only by snowcat, areas with the longest vertical descents of any resort in North America. We knew from experience there was world-class powder. Steep and deep. Time to get my snorkel out for ski pictures that would drive the hard cores back home crazy.

The conditions were just what we'd hoped for. High, vertical runs with fresh, light, perfect powder. I pushed myself hard, enjoying the air in my lungs, the strength that surged through me once again. I had to be careful as poling with my right arm seemed to cause a slight swelling of the right breast. I had been warned by the radiation oncologist that if that happened, the measurements and co-ordinates taken and fed to the computer would be off course. They would need to start again by re-simulating and then waiting another nine days to start treatment.

Okay, so now you're shaking your head and asking why I was tempting fate like that. Didn't I want to get this over with? Wasn't I scared of causing a setback?

In my defence, I can only say that *powder* skiing is one of the softest ski-poling sports out there. You plant in virtual air. I was careful not to use the right arm to push myself when traversing or walking uphill. My left arm was strong enough to compensate. Add to that my determination and downright donkeyness to continue doing what I placed above almost everything else in my life and you had my reasons.

And . . . I should add there were those wonderful things called ice packs and anti-inflammatory drugs.

Whoever said "Money can't buy happiness" never experienced a deep, fresh-powder day on new boards! The Revelstoke ski shop had a sale where I bought my Salomon skis and a new jacket as well.

It snowed almost the entire trip so by the third day we got the untracked "pow" we were hoping for. It's what made living worthwhile, those moments when you couldn't get the grin off your face and all you could think to say was "Wahoo!" over and over. I was in heaven for not minutes but hours. The wheeziness in my chest only happened when I had to jump turn the steepest slopes. I was careful to take breaks until I caught my breath again. The energy level was at an all-time high and I was determined to make the most of it.

Sadly, before we knew it, we were back in Kelowna awaiting my first encounter with the radiation beam. I can't say I was looking forward to it, not like I had for the chemo. Once I decided I needed it, you couldn't get the chemo into me fast enough. But I had been through so much; I was feeling great and the thought of going backwards was enough to make me squeeze the stuffing out of Homer. Kim's poor little bear was getting thinner every day.

After a hot soak in my uncle's tub I stood to reach for a towel and caught a full-length glimpse of myself in the mirror. I hadn't looked at myself in ages. I mean really looked at myself. It was shocking! Why was my right breast half deflated and twisting off to one side with a bright pink incision mark above it? The new scar cinched in the surrounding tissue, which made a roll of what looked like fat spill over it. I was so white and doughy-looking. I had lost a lot of my muscle mass while parked on that couch all those weeks.

This was my first full-on eyeful; I hadn't stopped to assess the damage since before the surgeries. Silly, I know, but I just never wanted to look too closely at myself, knowing I might not like what I saw. And I had been right. There was a frightening resemblance to my mother's decaying body before she died. A storm of panic gathered somewhere behind my eyes. Was I dying?

I looked up. My face was blotchy from steam and my hairless features enhanced every deep wrinkle and crevice. My head was a bowling ball covered in little black patches of hair. I had a cowhide head!

I couldn't look anymore. I was disgusting! Before I could stop it, a deep desolation descended upon me, threatening to carry me fast and far away. My face contorted grotesquely and I bent over, the weight of the shock almost too much to bear.

I was a freak. A flipping freak! Why hadn't I been warned that I would look like this?

And worse, how could I *live* like this?

I faced the mirror again, thinking I was possibly overreacting. Nope.

My self-image shattered. Like Humpty Dumpty I was merely shards on the floor. Ugly bits of what I used to be. I hammered myself with disgusting phrases I had heard on the school ground while hanging around malicious little girls.

"You're revolting. You look like a monster. Get away from us, you freak."

I *was* a freak. I looked back and stared hard at the mirror.

Who is that poor wretched soul? Please, tell me that is not me. Please.

How had it come to this? What had happened? Where was my body?

A burst of bawling worsened the image with swollen, red-rimmed eyes, runny nose and graceless grimace. It was amidst this catastrophic breakdown that my brain threw me a lifeline, a pleasant memory floating to the surface.

My reflection in the mirror melted away and I was once again riding the T-bar on a snowy mountainside with the good-looking Dr. Y beside me. His mouth opens and I hear his words, loud and clear.

" . . . because you are. You're beautiful."

Lyrics from a popular song popped into my head, "You're beautiful, you're beautiful, it's true," and I chanted this to myself a few times. It seemed to work. The monster in the mirror faded away and instead, I saw a transformed Cinderella being appraised from afar by the Don Juan of Dentists.

The vapor of nastiness evaporated and all seemed right once again. The moment passed and, like the Grinch's heart, mine grew from pea-size to normal in a matter of seconds. All because someone I admired still thought I was beautiful enough to tell me so. It was something all my friends and husband, with the best intentions, could say to me until blue in the face but I would never believe it. They had a habit of saying whatever they thought I needed to hear. It was called false reassurance and I hated it. But Dr. Y was different. He genuinely meant what he'd said. His eyes couldn't lie that convincingly. For whatever reason, Dr. Y thought I was beautiful. I believed that and it was enough to pull me up. Way up. I wiped my face dry with the back of my hand, high-fived the disfigured woman in the mirror and left the bathroom with a smile on my distorted, mottled face.

The following day when Homer, Barry and I arrived at the clinic for my first radiation treatment I was an apprehensive mess. It was such a mind screw . . . to feel so alive and then subject yourself to something you knew would take at least some of that joie de vivre away. I was confident I had prepared myself. I had taken all the vitamins and protective herbs recommended by the naturopath and had remained active each and every day. I was ready to receive as much radiation as they dared without damaging too many healthy cells, but each treatment came with risks and you wondered if you would be the one-in-a-thousand that grew a third arm. I worried I would flinch at the wrong time, causing the radiation beam to hit my heart, pierce my lung or scar me forever. So much had gone sideways that I couldn't relax. There was nothing I would trust.

So, I am sorry to report, there were big alligator tears that coursed down my cheeks as I lay beneath that daunting machine with my right arm twisted high behind my head. Breast bared. Whirring noises. Clicks. All alone. The techs line you up and then leave you, returning to a hidden control room, looking at you through a camera. I felt like I was at the bottom of a tall barrel. I wanted my mother. I wanted an ice cream cone. I wanted whatever it was that would make all of this go away. I stuck my tongue out at the large rotating laser head as it passed in front of the camera. If the techs had noticed, they never said a word on their return.

I was the immature expression of a clipped wild turkey. I needed my normal life back and to do that, I had to lie on that metal stretcher and let that scary Wizard of Oz contraption do what it could for me, 15 more times.

Hang in there, Deb. You can do this.

Twenty minutes later I was told I was finished for the week. See you on Monday. It must have gone okay? No one said anything to the contrary. After jumping off the steel gurney, I readjusted my hospital clothes and hurried to the change rooms. You didn't have to tell me twice to get out of there. Just being in that building with all that radiation flying around gave me the heebie-jeebies. Peaceful piano music or not.

Back at my uncle's house, with a small glass of red wine in front of me, I tried to shake off the funk. I reached for Homer, hugging him tightly, and took a sip of wine. I swirled the warm liquid in my mouth but it didn't go down well. The guilt of running back to an old habit, of self-medicating, ruined the taste and I pushed the glass aside. Wasn't alcohol the number one suspect in what had put me here in the first place? If I didn't change my ways, wouldn't I risk having to do all of this again? The thought made me tired. I dragged myself and Homer upstairs for a nap.

My weekend was treatment-free. That would be enough time to pull myself back out of the pit I had fallen into. One treat at a time. I was thinking a shrimp stir-fry, a ready-made salad and a movie. Sometimes it's easy to divert the attention-disordered.

12

Radiation Meets ADD and Drama

Now that I was in the system and had received my first radiation treatment, the remaining time in Kelowna was like a work schedule. My weeks would begin on Monday. I received a little blue card with my name and clinic number on it. Inside the card were written the dates and times for the next week of treatments. They ranged from 8:48 a.m. to 4:26 p.m. weekdays. Some days there were two times penciled in, meaning I was to see the radiologist as well.

We placed our parking pass on the Suburban's dash. It seemed like such a small lot for all of the people coming and going but there always seemed to be a spot. Some days I opted to walk or jog. It depended on the weather or how tired I was.

At first it was tricky remembering to bring my hospital gowns each time. It felt more like an outing. "Just popping down to the cancer unit, dear. Back in an hour."

After reading the book *Crazy Sexy Cancer Tips* by Kris Carr, I contemplated attaching lace and rhinestones to the drab blue gowns. They were dowdy enough to deflate the cheeriest soul. But thinking about it was a chore in itself. My energy was definitely starting to wane as the treatments continued.

Once inside the cancer clinic, I headed down "radiation alley," passing stations named The Cabin, The Lake, The Park and arriving at The Hills with mere minutes to spare. I placed my little blue card in the drop-off slot at an unmanned desk. Eventually someone would notice the card and know I had arrived.

I changed in the room across from my station and then took my street clothes with me to the waiting area. There was a jigsaw puzzle started on the table, stacks of magazines, a water fountain and a blanket warmer. At -20°C outside and without hair, I was tempted more than once to crawl right inside the warmer.

One journal entry mentioned I was cranky and not in the mood for the cold fingers of the radiation technicians as they pulled my torso this way and pushed my butt that way to line up their co-ordinates. They marked on my skin with a felt pen each time I came. There was a green lighted line I could see mirrored in the head of the radiation machine that ran from beneath my armpit down along my body. That particular day there was a young man joining the usual two young women working on me. I made a face at having to bare myself yet again to another male and wondered at my childishness. It was just another mutilated old-lady-boob to him.

My arm was stretched over my head, the points lined up and they all left the room. The machine whirred and beeped, then after a few minutes it moved to the other side of my body where it repeated the process of noises. When the techs returned I was already sitting up, re-draping myself, and trying to get off the steel slab.

"See you tomorrow," I called out, like it was a job. That cracked me up.

I was a fragile statement in need of comic relief.

Back in the change room I removed my gowns and slathered the breast area with a thick cream the specialists recommended I bring for each visit. The skin was warm beneath my fingers and would continue to heat up throughout the day. The cream cooled the radiated area and helped prevent blistering. Actually, the heat didn't feel bad, it being January and all; like putting a pocket warmer in your bra.

I got dressed and walked to The Hills reception cubicle where my little blue card was now in the pick-up slot. Still no one seated at the desk.

I was done for the day but the technicians had only started. I wondered how they felt about the never-ending stream of people battling cancer. Old ones, young ones. Ones that arrived in wheelchairs or jogged in like I had. I came to the conclusion it was not an easy job for any of us.

Finally, there was a light at the end of the long tunnel; only seven more treatments to go. The shopping bug had died off but the sales had been incredible. I was currently on official notice with my husband and the credit card company. But yes, thanks, honey, I did feel much better with a new teal-coloured fleece shirt that complimented the grey on my head. Everything else I owned made me look dead when I wasn't wearing a wig or a bright scarf.

After a solid week of radiation treatments, my brother Danny came to visit. He drove from Invermere through a blinding snowstorm and showed up at the Pheasant and Quail Pub for the Super Bowl game where (*yes!*) I did win a door prize, free appetizers and the entire football pool for the night. It was more than enough money to buy all our food and drinks for the evening. Wasn't my mother amazing? She seemed to have a lot of pull from wherever she was at.

The three of us caught Big White's fresh powder on Monday after a spectacular dump of overnight snow. We ended up exhausted but happy.

After my Tuesday treatment we toured wineries for the day. I didn't mind being the designated driver. It was the beginning of the new me. Best get used to it sooner than later.

That night I cooked a special dinner of spruce grouse, complete with homemade chutney and trimmings, in celebration of my brother's 52nd birthday. We didn't get a chance to celebrate our birthdays together very often so I added a death-by-chocolate cake to the menu. It was so special that Danny had come to see how I was doing.

Things were going well. The radiation was causing some pins and needles in my breast but my energy was still respectable and the moods manageable. Hot flashes continued on a regular basis, especially when I was grumpy. They acted as a shock collar, forcing me to calm down whenever I got really angry. Barry was still giving me a fairly wide berth although my uncle's roomy home felt very small some days.

Saying goodbye to my brother was hard. He had places to go, people to see. He left me with a bag of hulled hemp seeds, a "superfood," he called them. I had no idea what that meant but I put the bag into the box of groceries we had brought from home and forgot about it. Turns out hemp seeds are high in protein and extremely healthy for you. A superfood means something that has more than one unique beneficial property to it. Now I eat hemp seeds before or after a workout to help replenish my body. I think of Danny every time.

For Valentine's Day Barry bought me some ski poles to go with the new mitts he got me for Christmas. The mitts were too big to put through the wrist straps on poles I'd been using since 1970-something. I said the poles would make a great Valentine's gift, as indeed they did. No flowers and especially no chocolates were needed. I hoped to be leaving Kelowna, headed home in five days, so the flowers would go to waste.

We did, however, decide to go out for a special dinner. Because I could be fussy (Barry's words, not mine), I was in charge of where to go. Someone recommended the Yellowhouse Restaurant, using words like gourmet, delightful, and seafood. I called in the reservation a day early.

Valentine's Day came and we stood in the entranceway of the Yellowhouse dressed in our finery. We looked fabulous but our faces were flushed from an argument over where to park. A waitress laden with heaped salad plates walked by and we were astonished to recognize her. It was Meghan, a friend's daughter. What a pleasant surprise. This was going to be a fun night!

Fun . . . until they couldn't find our reservation on one of the busiest nights of the year. As fate goes, I had accidentally made a reservation at the Yang Japanese House, the phone number listed above the Yellowhouse in the phone directory. Did radiation affect one's eyesight? Nice try, Deb.

We looked at each other as people tried to squeeze past us to their cozy seats, then headed outside, away from the warmth, the ambience, the intoxicating smells of infused sauces and swirled delights. Neither of us wanted to eat Japanese fare, not with our hearts set on candlelight and croquettes. A second, bigger argument ensued.

"I told you to re-check the reservation this morning," he fired at the back of my head.

"Who the (heck) rechecks a reservation?" I countered. Sheesh. I stomped off but he followed.

And yes, he brought up the cell phone I lost two days ago, the carpet that I ruined cleaning with bleach in our bedroom at home and the $2,000 worth of deck sealant I applied that bubbled up and flaked off. Why wouldn't I do what he said? He was the voice of reason, of common sense. I paid no attention to details. When would I start listening?

"I *am* listening," I hollered for the 10,000th time in my life. "I just don't *agree!*" Especially when my translation of his words was "You're a wing nut, a wing nut, a wing nut."

I drove too fast on the way home, almost had an accident, and felt like bashing the Suburban through my uncle's garage door. I huffed up the stairs, shouted some more as I undressed and flung my wig against a wall where it plopped down out of sight. No wig stand for it tonight. No makeup remover. No teeth brushed. I went to bed. It was 7:45.

I spent Valentine's evening trying to draw some comfort from a perplexed but quiet Homer. I ate the emergency-only chocolate bar from the bottom of my purse, cramming half of it into my face in one shot. It was so old it tasted like pocket fluff.

I didn't hear Barry when he came to bed hours later. I did smell the wine. I wondered if he noticed chocolate on *my* breath. At that moment I didn't care if he noticed. I wouldn't have cared if it had been *his* chocolate bar he'd bought for millions at an auction. (If there is such a thing?)

By morning I could see it was all so *us* and thinking the whole absurdity took another week off my life. Why did everything have to be so stressful? Why couldn't we simply laugh at all of these screw-ups and just keep going? Why did Barry think he could fix me? Was this a cancer treatment problem or was I going to be like this the rest of my life? Well, I *had* been almost like this for 50 years and you know what? It didn't really bother me. Too bad it bothered someone else so much.

If only I could find that darned cell phone (and my missing gloves and my watch)! Then maybe I'd have a half a leg to stand on in the trust department. I knew I wasn't crazy but things were adding up against me.

Incredible highs and the bottom-of-the-barrel lows are a definite symptom of ADD. I have felt my skin vibrate with joy as I drove to the ski hill on a sunny day. Then, just days later, I'd be weeping, overwhelmed with feelings of futility. But when you're in that top moment the world sparkles and it was in that space I jogged to the Cancer Centre of the Southern Interior for my last radiation treatment on February 18. Indeed, the final treatment of this entire, horrific roller coaster ride.

I jogged not because I had a ton of energy. I didn't. It had been declining steadily with the treatments. I jogged because I was making a statement to myself. I had cancer but it did not beat me. I made it through alive and in one piece. I had one and a half breasts, five scars, a head of grey peach fuzz and nothing but the rest of an amazing, never-a-dull-moment life to look forward to. The suffering had ended, hopefully forever.

I was now officially a breast cancer survivor and would be until I died . . . hopefully not from cancer because then I wouldn't have been a survivor after all. In fact, being called a survivor should mean I survived the treatment regimens and nothing more. I would be foolish to think I survived cancer. We had thrown almost everything in the arsenal at it. But now we had to wait and see what happened. Whatever. I was out the other side and still breathing.

Three streets from my uncle's house on the homeward jog I slowed to a walk because I could no longer stop the flood of emotion overwhelming me. Inside my head a movie was playing, showing the momentous single moments of the entire cancer experience. Through unstoppable tears I saw everything: the love, the pain, the calls, the concern, the small triumphs, the harsh realities, the rug being pulled out beneath my feet over and over, the shock on Barry's face, the shock on Sharon's face, on Sandi's, the arms that held me, the tears that mingled with mine, the strong hands that soothed me, relaxed me, comforted me. The parade of people — some I've mentioned, many I haven't — Drs. V, Y, P, Q, R, KJ, H, Z and our families and the e-mails from old friends, the staff at all the offices, clinics and hospitals. I made it to my uncle's home, being sure to thank all the folks who stopped to see if I was okay.

I walked in the door where my husband stood looking awkward and uncertain.

"Is it over?" he asked.

"I hope so," I said, my face red and puffy from crying.

I wrapped my arms around him and we cried together. It was then I realized how much Barry had been holding in. He hadn't been welcomed to voice an opinion or even a concern for the past seven months. I was worried he would say the wrong thing and send me into a tailspin. It had happened before and I had refused to risk it happening at this worst time of my life. Yet I was perpetually mad at him for not saying the *right* things. The truth was I wouldn't let him in close enough to say anything. I never once stopped to think maybe it was the worst time of his life too. Our tears flowed because this had happened not just to me but to us. We cried for what we'd been through, for the uncertainty of the future and because the worst was hopefully behind us. I have never loved my husband more than I did at that very moment.

Relief, affection, sadness, tiredness, hope and willpower flowed through me. It was time to take all the hard memories of the past year and move them as far from my present thoughts as possible.

The cancerous chains were off and I was flying again. I wanted to relish this ecstasy for as long as I could hang onto it. We started the celebration with dinner at the classy Yellowhouse Restaurant. I bought a new outfit and put on the blonde wig. Barry couldn't take his eyes off me as I came down the stairs. Now that was the right way to start a celebratory evening. I never said a word about where he parked this time. And *he* phoned in the reservation.

We had the night of our lives! And Meghan, the waitress we knew, and her boyfriend joined us for dessert, something that would not have happened while she was working on Valentine's Day. We returned home after winning some money at the casino, got undressed, cleaned up, and crawled into bed. Not even one argument.

"I guess we weren't meant to have dinner there on Valentine's Day, after all," I said.

Barry reached over to stroke my head. "You're so beautiful," he said as we wandered off to sleep.

By the end of February 2011, I had been scanned, probed, needled, cut, reopened, re-cut, poisoned and nuked. The scars were fading to a less angry colour of pink and the burnt radiated skin was turning to tan. It was time for my body to rest and heal and let the world of pharmaceuticals protect me from a big-C recurrence.

I was on tamoxifen, one pill a day for the next five years. Some forms of breast cancer, like mine, are hormone receptor positive. This means estrogen and progesterone can be used by cancer cells to grow. Tamoxifen blocks this process and thus inhibits cancer cell growth. Side effects are extremely menopausal sounding — weight gain, hot flashes, loss of libido, tiredness, aching joints, hair thinning (*not again!*) and headaches.

Tamoxifen can also increase the risk for uterine cancer. That thought rattled me but until I reached menopause, and quit producing estrogen and progesterone, there didn't seem to be an alternative. Sandi assured me that when I did reach menopause I could switch to safer alternatives.

As an added precaution, because I was spared the last two chemo treatments, I was being injected once a month with a second anti-cancer drug called Zoladex. It would decrease the amount of estrogen and progesterone that my body produced. Side effects? Even more hot flashing, tiredness, decreased libido and weight gain. My waistline was doomed!

Good thing I still had a cute butt. Oh wait . . . I wouldn't care because I would lose my sex drive. Maybe we should put husbands on the same stuff at the same time?

13

Detoxing

Back in the Bulkley Valley we resumed our normal whirlwind life, spending half the week in Houston and half at our place on the ski hill. Every Wednesday we stuffed four 75-litre packs with food, clothes and other essentials, drove an hour to the hill, then marched the packs up a snowy trail to our log cabin on Hudson Bay Mountain. We started the fire in the cabin's wood burner before returning to the vehicle to grab another load.

The cabin sits about 1650 metres above sea level so getting to it ensures a good cardiopulmonary workout. I reminded myself all that oxygen was great for killing cancer cells. I know I should have felt confident I could relax a bit after surgery, chemo and radiation, but letting go of the fear did not come easy. I knew those cancer cells hated oxygen so I volunteered to make a third trip to move our vehicle from the unloading zone to the parking lot below. That meant another climb back to the cabin. I felt my softened muscles scream as they turned from marshmallow back to steel. Well . . . maybe stiff cardboard.

When I returned the cabin was warm enough to unpack the lettuce and cucumbers into the propane fridge. It would be another two hours before we could relax comfortably without our coats and boots on.

Then the socializing began. Thrilling Thursday at the main ski lodge, with free appys and draws for goodies, started at 4 p.m. so we tromped down and surprised the bar staff. There were hugs all around but I did cause an eyebrow or two to be raised when I ordered a soda water with ice and a splash of white grape juice. It's a friend's recipe called a Saudi Champagne and it rescued me from my old habits. There were three of us on the ski hill that year that went through breast cancer at the exact same time. The other two still drink alcohol but I wasn't ready to go back there. That's not saying I didn't leap off the wagon occasionally, but I kept reminding myself that "There is no set amount of alcohol that has been determined to be safe" once you've been diagnosed with breast cancer, especially estrogen-fed cancers like mine.

Friday and Saturday we socialized at other cabins and on Sunday we skied all day before loading everything — spent battery packs, empty beverage bottles, water jugs, laundry, leftover food, garbage — back into the packs for the return journey. In the summer we do the exact same thing at a cabin on a lake. Load, unload, reload and re-unload. It's a lifestyle choice, complete with gas lamps and outhouses at both properties. It keeps us busy and healthy.

So how did I get cancer? Was it the premenopausal hormonal imbalance? Before my diagnosis I could go from a happy Care Bear to a dragon with a sore tooth in record speed. My periods were drying up and becoming sporadic events. On top of that, I consumed immoderate quantities of alcohol and chocolate, not to mention a weakness for fatty chicken wings and salty Chinese food. Add a lifetime of hair and skin product toxins, BBQ charred meat and vegetables, suntanning at a salon before annual trips south, the stress of living with a Gemini (when you are an ADD Sagittarian) and a Suburban-wrecking MVA and you had a recipe for breast cancer. I had no doubt that's how it happened. It wasn't just one thing. I had bought a lot of tickets in the cancer lottery and finally won.

My life was spared, thanks to an early diagnosis, but some are not. Months into my cancer journey Sandi visited our ski cabin. She arrived with what looked like the weight of the world on her shoulders. After questioning her, she admitted she had "lost another patient to breast cancer" that day.

I recall my eyes went wide and my mouth dropped open. "What? People still die from breast cancer?"

It was her turn to look surprised. Hadn't I known that all along?

Okay, that got my attention. I figured everyone had it cut out and nuked before sweeping the issue under their carpet, like I had. I knew my life expectancy had been tampered with, but to die from breast cancer? Couldn't they catch everyone's early now that they had the capability?

Well no. It appears not everyone self-examines their breasts, goes for mammograms or makes appointments to see a doctor when there's a concern. They don't always catch cancer early enough and even an early diagnosis doesn't guarantee a cure.

What did I know? You had to hit me over the head with an IV pole sometimes.

Now that we were home, trying to catch up with even my closest friends and family seemed next to impossible. I called people with the phone tilted to my ear as I chopped, stirred, folded clothes, researched the Internet or dusted (in that order). No wonder I was so tired! I literally crashed, flopping to the couch or bed between tasks, not able to muster enough energy to get up for a glass of water.

Ridiculous. When would I learn to slow down? Then again, I bought a card for a friend's 60th that said to "Live it up now. You can rest when you're dead." Maybe that's what the go-go-go was all about? Somewhere deep down I worried about dying with a list of regrets. Things like learning how to type with 10 fingers or say more than "Two fish tacos, please" in Spanish.

I didn't think it was completely that. It was also about trying to get back to my normal life, and not having enough energy to get there . . . yet.

Toward the end of March, Barry and I pulled out a bottle of Veuve Clicquot Ponsardin, delicious champagne given to us by a friend at the start of our cancer journey. Himself a cancer survivor, the donor wanted us to use it to celebrate the end of the treatment ordeal.

Was I ready? I knew Barry was and so I suggested he get it out. I enjoyed a few commemorative sips to assure myself I was (almost) back to normal. If I said it enough, maybe it would be so? No matter, my husband deserved being thanked and congratulated for surviving as well.

"So," I said, after clinking glasses, "how many more years are you in for?"

"Are you implying our marriage is like a prison sentence?"

"Yeh, what are you in for?"

"What I'm in for," he said, grabbing me and swinging me around, "is keeping that smile on your face. Any chance of that?"

I laughed. "Only if you keep bringing me lattes when I need them the most."

I tried to look serious. "Sure you want to keep doing this? This might not be the end, you know."

"As long as you and your chemo-brain don't burn the house down around us, I'll stay. In fact, I'm going to hang around to make sure that doesn't happen. I'm your personal prison guard. So now who's in jail?"

"Sign me up," I said. "You're hired and you have a job with me for as long as you want."

I still tired easily with exertion, especially when Sandi and I ran our usual 40 minutes through Houston or when I swam at the pool. I needed a nap after those excursions or I wouldn't last the day.

The side scars from the lymph node removal and the drainage tube still bothered me. It was like I had a second armpit; the indentation was quite pronounced. I booked another appointment with Robin, the massage therapist, who manipulated the skin around the scar to loosen the adhesions. The movement was better but the area still ached after a day of skiing or when I stretched out my arm at the pool. The numbness between my shoulder and elbow was less and, even better, the semi-depression of the past month seemed to be lifting.

Emerging from cancer treatment is not easy. You now have time to face everything that happened, to look at yourself in the mirror and re-evaluate. I had to forgive my old self, accept my new self and face the fact that this might not be finished, that there might be a relapse, a new primary tumour or side effects from my current drugs. It's called "survivorship," an emotional process of shedding the old skin and getting comfortable in the new one. I think that definitely deserved a bit of champagne.

The treatments ended February 18th but the saga continued. I settled into life on the drug tamoxifen quite nicely. Other than the bi-hourly hot flash my mood had improved, my energy level was climbing and my long lost libido wandered in from the pasture.

It took four months to grow one inch of grey hair on the top of my head. At first I thought the grey was a result of treatment but then I realized I'd been dying the colour back into it since I'd been 40-something. Grey was now my new "natural" colour. Sigh.

And then it started to curl. My hair was usually straight as a ski pole but now it had baby curls like we made with bobby pins when we were kids. Yes, I used to pay big money to get permed, curly hair, but not this kind! To tell you the truth, more than anything my locks reminded me of pubic hair! There, I said it. It was thick, coarse, and curly. I was tempted to shave it off again.

But I had to admit I was warmer with than without it. When you get older warmth is one of the main things a woman wants, along with love, food, security and someone (who does everything her way) with whom to grow old. I did, however, still reach for a hat when I made a run to the outhouse in the middle of the night at the ski hill. Not because someone might see me, but because it got cold!

Now that there was colour, albeit the wrong one, atop my head, some of my girlfriends tried to get me to lose the wig/ball cap/ kerchief/doily. "Okay," I said, "as long as you sit with me in the lounge with *your* grey hair shining through." We all spent hundreds of dollars a year covering up the fact that we had grey and white roots, that we were aging. So why would anyone figure it would be okay to flash it now?

Anyway, I fully intended to get it dyed as soon as the medical world permitted. My books said six months and to use an ammonia-free solution. My friend said two months so I was going with her. Maybe I should have kept asking for someone to say one month?

I had questioned my oncologists about performing a detoxification right after my treatments ended but neither felt it was mandatory. Regardless, there were hordes of information on the Internet and in health food stores that said otherwise. I figured, what could it hurt?

My organs and skin had been exposed to some extremely traumatizing elements. Between the chemo, radiation and who knows what with the anesthetics and surgeries, I could only assume there might be some benefit in a good cleansing. After the CT scans and 16 radiation treatments, I was amazed I didn't glow in the dark.

A huge part of survivorship is worrying about and doing something to prevent, or at least detect early, a recurrence. When I called to make an appointment for the breast thermal imaging (looking for hot spots that might hint at a recurrence) at the Finlandia Pharmacy in Vancouver, the clinician suggested I soak for an hour in two kilos of aluminum-free baking soda and two kilos of sea salt mixed in a warm bath to help neutralize the effects of all that radiation.

Barry rolled his eyes to the ceiling and then wondered if our septic field would survive. I worried my skin would turn even whiter. I already looked like a snow goose but was determined not to use the (carcinogenic) tanning booths before our upcoming end-of-treatment holiday.

I soaked without incident and it felt good enough to do it weekly for a month. As I said, what harm? My skin felt smoother and that was a bonus. The second thing I did to detox was omit dairy, processed foods and wheat from my diet, limit sugar to absolute necessity for 30 days and flush my system with a lakeful of green tea.

I took cleansing capsules purchased from the health food store first thing in the morning and then right before I went to bed. The advertising says the capsules cleanse "the entire body" and my morning ablutions proved it!

I was flushing the pills down with a quart of organic apple juice. Apple juice and apple cider vinegar have long been used as a natural liver detox program. You can Google this and get a three-day regime to follow; one includes nothing but juice and vinegar. That was a bit too intense for me. I wasn't going to inflict any more pain than necessary for a good long while. Enough was enough already.

The final part of my detox plan was three one-hour infrared sauna sessions. Different from traditional saunas that heat the body from the outside in, these saunas let the body absorb the safe light waves which break down the congested fatty or water tissues, where the majority of collected toxins, acids, pathogens and carcinogens are stored. So instead of sweating out 2–3 percent of the stored toxins, you release up to 20 percent. A bit of damage control after what had been done to my body lately.

My friends set the heat on theirs at 100°F and it rose gradually to 120°F while I sat inside and sweated enough to ring out a washcloth. I brought my Gregorian chants CD and listened to a Divine Light Invocation. Might as well purify my mind as well as my body. They say a healthy mental state is as important as a healthy body.

Lots of exercise always soothed me so I started a more regular routine at the pool and gym. I tried to do something physically challenging for 40 minutes every day. In the evenings I forced myself to sit in front of a candle, trying to clear my mind. It never worked; my mind always went 100 miles an hour but my legs felt relaxed. That was something.

At the end of the week I noticed my skin felt silky smooth and I had more energy than in the previous month. That might have been from the detox and/or the new vitamin plan I started once the radiation ended — a woman's multivitamin, fish oil, green tea extract, vitamin E, Bone-Up for calcium, a multi B for nerves and extra vitamin D because we don't get a lot of sun exposure in northwest B.C. Also, vitamin D has been linked to cancer prevention. I swirled a teaspoon of a greens concentrate extract with added antioxidants into a quarter cup of water every morning to balance my pH levels and I still drank the juice of half a lemon in my herbal tea. I ate my oatmeal with blueberry yogurt and freshly ground flax seeds. (Then I brushed my teeth. Lemon juice is supposedly hard on tooth enamel.)

My plan was to maintain this regime for the five years I was on the tamoxifen, if not for the rest of my life. Practical or not, I was helping myself. And that did wonders for my peace of mind.

14

Hot Boobs

From what I'd read, it was as important to feed your soul as it was to nurture your body. Stress is a risk factor for cancer, as is smoking and excessive drinking. Lots of us self-medicate with alcohol, which is like putting out a fire with gasoline.

Changing what you put into your body is your first line of defence against cancer. The second is putting good things into your mind. Things like stillness and serenity. Relaxation techniques to bring you back to zero, to stop the incessant roar of life for a spell. Learning to relax is not an easy thing for someone with ADD, but at this stage of my life it was important. My friends recommended yoga, stretching, Pilates, tai chi, ballroom dancing and swimming.

If ever there was a time to reward myself for all that I'd survived, it was now. Say thanks to my mind and body for not giving up. For fighting as hard as they had. It would be fun and healthy. At least, that's what I told myself.

There are plenty of ways to pat yourself on the back. It might be as simple as buying a commemorative item — jewellery, a piece of clothing, a special picture framed. Treat yourself to a spa-day or host one at home with friends, go camping, plan a romantic night somewhere special or throw a girl's night-in. Pizza, toe-painting and comparing notes about the habits of males could be good for a giggle.

For us, we decided Costa Rica would be the prize at the bottom of the Cracker Jack box — long beaches, pure drinking water, stunning mountains and rejuvenating, volcano-warmed hot springs. Chemo patient detox central. Countdown to departure, three months.

Now that cancer was on the back burner I was able to focus on the whiplash from the November 2009 accident. The ICBC settlement for my neck injuries came through. My son jokingly advised me to put it all on black at a casino. I did almost the same thing. I invested the money in the stock market. After carefully choosing two recommended stocks from advisors on BNN's *Market Place*, I waited only 16 days and cleared $10,000. Good enough for me! I again thanked my mom, sold the stocks, then rubbed my hands together and said to an astonished Barry, "That's how you play the stock market." I could now pay for whiplash treatments *and* a trip to Costa Rica.

Our adventure began with a flight from Smithers to Vancouver, where we had a 10-hour stopover. I planned to use part of that time in front of the breast thermal imaging machine at the Finlandia Pharmacy. I know . . . I know . . . it's a controversial test and should never be used as a substitute for mammograms. In fact, at Finlandia, you must sign a form saying you realize this test should never be used as an alternative to mammograms.

According to the literature I read, thermal imaging is done with a special infrared camera that maps your hot and cold spots. It's based on the premise that precancerous and cancerous tissue creates heat as it increases circulation to the cells. Did you know a cancerous tumour can hold open blood vessels, reopen dormant vessels and, even worse, create new ones to feed an insatiable need for nutrients?

Sophisticated computers are used to detect these temperature variations and produce high resolution images. These images are used to alert your regular physician to possible irregularities in the breast. And the best part, there's no radiation involved.

My plan was to use it once a year between my annual mammos or MRIs. You do have to pay for it. It's a private service but one highly recommended for people wanting a test between tests or to see things from a different angle. For me, it was a part of survivorship.

The procedure started in a small private room in a building across the street from the pharmacy. While facing the thermal imaging camera, I was asked to strip to my waist and instructed on how to pose, arms over head in five different positions. My own erotica for Barry. Good enough for an upcoming birthday gift, although the final photos were very psychedelic in greens, oranges and reds. He loved them.

I was very emotional during the entire procedure; possibly because I worried they would find something. Over the past year every test I took seemed to end with more bad news. I was like the dog cowering at the sight of a raised broom.

We finished the photo session and I redressed. The tech said the results would be mailed to me. I explained I would not be home for three weeks and would be holding my breath the whole time. We compromised. When she received the results, before mailing them out, the tech would read them and send me an e-mail. It turned out to be a silly arrangement. It almost ruined our holiday.

We arrived in Costa Rica April 13 in the morning. My eyes were crossed from lack of sleep and a large kink had formed in my neck. Heat slammed into me as I descended from the plane at San Jose. "Bring it on," I thought. "Hit me harder. I dare you."

Like sheeple, we obligingly followed our fellow travellers through the immigration lineup to our suitcases and then to a lineup of taxi and shuttle drivers waving sheets of paper with names written on them. Our name was scrawled on one such flag. We placed ourselves into the fine care of Jose from Heredia, who packed us off to his hotel for the next two nights. We whizzed past palm trees, flowering bushes and signs written in Spanish. A flood of words from past trips to Mexico came back to me. *¿Dónde está el baño?*

Jose was a savvy guide. He directed us to the university quarter for cheap *cervezas* (beers) and *ceviche mariscos* (raw seafood marinated in fresh limes, spices and onion). We sat for hours watching the hustle and bustle of San Jose until the sun went down. Giddy from exhaustion and a few sips of Barry's Coronas, I exhaled deeply. I had been holding my breath for nine long months.

The following day we toured a coffee plantation, a waterfall park with a zoo filled with long, nasty snakes, poisonous frogs and white-faced monkeys, and the highlight . . . a hike to the actively smoking Poás Volcano. This was a dangerous and exciting country.

That night I found an e-mail from the technician at the Finlandia Pharmacy. The results had come back. I didn't realize I was not breathing until I read the words "Please be advised that you should contact your doctor as soon as possible." The air trapped in my lungs came out in a loud "Ooof" like I had been hit in the gut with a baseball bat. I bent over for a second, wondering if I was going to throw up.

It passed. My brain started hollering, "I knew it, I *knew* it! This isn't over. The nightmare continues."

I fired off an e-mail to Sandi on the hotel computer. It read "Panic, panic, freak-out, distressed, overstressed, what now, why me, panicked and frightened. Love, Deb."

I then fell apart.

What did they find? Had the cancer spread? Was it in my bones, my brain, my organs? Would it be quick? Should I go home? Should I go to the hospital here? Would I have time for a shot of tequila? Do they have tequila in Costa Rica?

My husband thankfully pointed out I should calm down a bit, possibly with a glass of red wine in my hand? Stress caused cancer, remember? This was a holiday and the odd drink was not going to kill me. And even if it did, at least I'd be happy.

He was trying to get a smile out of me.

It took more than a glass to get that smile.

Okay. Back to the world of having cancer. So what was I afraid of? They'd already put me through everything they could dream up, except a torture rack, which maybe came next. So I'd be taller and thinner. Nothing wrong with that.

Come on, Deb. This could be dealt with. Just another round of cut, poison and nuke. I could do this. I *would* do this. I absolutely refused to exit this life before I had grandkids. At the rate our kids were moving, that could take another full lifetime. We would just deal with it. I had enough energy to kick some more cancer butt! Didn't I?

Look at the positive side. Here was another license to eat sympathy chocolate again. Fighting for my life allowed me extra privileges. And just like that, as I prepared to hit the mini *super mercado* for a cart full of chocolate, a message appeared from Sandi. It was like she was in the room wrapping her arms around me and whispering, "Shhh, shhh, it will all be okay." She said any results from the imaging company were not a diagnosis. Only a biopsy after a mammo, an ultrasound or an MRI could give me that. And there were lots of false negatives and positives with thermal imaging, not to mention my breasts were still healing from surgeries and radiation. Healing promotes rapid cell growth, which would look similar to a cancer growth. She guaranteed me an appointment after my holiday and said she was *sure* there wouldn't be a recurrence this soon. Her words set me at ease.

Breathe in, breathe out. Breathe in, breathe out. The chocolate remained on the store shelf, at least this time. Two days after returning to Canada, the thermal tests arrived in my mail box. I took them directly to Sandi who quickly read the comments. Yes, there were numerous hot spots, but those spots aligned exactly with the recent surgeries and radiation.

On my next trip to Finlandia, someone new was running the program.

15

The Pot of Gold Called Costa Rica

Costa Rica was a fine country, extremely laid back. We never saw one calendar, only a few people wearing watches and even fewer computers. We had come to put the past nine months behind us, to regain strength, renew our spirits. So we relaxed, ate, swam, hiked, thought, remembered, cried, mopped up and came out eager to get back to simply living.

At the end of March, three weeks before travelling to Costa Rica, I started a second anti-cancer drug. It was called Zoladex and it stopped the production of estrogen (as opposed to the tamoxifen which blocked its absorption into cancer cells). It was a fingernail-sized, slow release pill that Sandi injected beneath the skin of my abdomen with a needle the size of a chop stick. It lasted a month and was then replaced. After a three-month trial I would graduate to a larger pill that lasted for three months. I didn't dare to imagine how big the three-month pill would be. Was my abdomen wide enough?

Before the first dose Sandi gave me some topical cream to apply at home over the injection site. It would numb the area, making the Zoladex injection more tolerable. I did as I was told, went to her office and changed into a hospital gown. When Sandi lifted the gown she saw a Band-Aid with big blobs of ointment still oozing out.

"How much did you use?" she asked.

"The whole tube. Why?" No, I hadn't read the instructions or asked my pharmacist how much to apply.

"That was enough for three injections," she said with a smirk.

Truth told, I was glad I had used it all because I never felt a thing.

Two days before our trip I received the second shot. No topical cream that time. I would take it as it came. Sandi gathered up the skin with her left hand but let go when I hollered, "Ow!"

She hadn't poked me with the needle yet.

My friend went and got a smaller needle full of anaesthetic. Once that was in I never felt anything but sheepish . . . which meant I jumped off the examination table, stuffing my shirt into my pants before Sandi had discarded the syringe.

"Wait. Don't you want a Band-Aid on that? It might continue to bleed for another minute or so."

"It's over. I'm okay," I said.

I can be such a hard-ass at times. Sandi knows that and didn't force the issue. I still haven't got the blood stains out of my shirt, underwear and blue jeans.

The initial reaction to Zoladex was extreme fatigue. I felt as if I hadn't slept in days and struggled to stay awake. The morning after receiving my shot I drove home and as soon as I reached the driveway and put the truck into park I sat for a minute. Before I knew it I was waking up. I had fallen asleep. Now that's scary!

The next thing to complain about was another drop in libido, which *was* a listed side effect. Of course that didn't last once in the land of palm trees, king-sized beds and half-naked bodies. It's not like I had anything against a roll on the beach. I just wasn't sure I could stay awake through the whole thing.

After two days in San Jose we took a gravel road off the main Costa Rican highway to our next resting spot, this time in the hills near the Arenal Volcano. The volcano was massive. It filled your vision, your head, your dreams and you couldn't stop looking at it. There had been no lava flow for six months but the people running our resort said it was only a matter of time. Our room wasn't ready so we got upgraded to the cabanas on the resort's highest ridge. The entire front of the room was glass and the volcano filled our view.

The bright green and blue parrots reminded me it was time to do something about the grey swirls atop my head; that and the fact that the room came with dark green and not the usual white towels which I took as a sign. A box of Clairol's Natural Instincts ammonia-free hair dye had been stowed in my suitcase for just such an occasion. By next morning a much younger (and happier) looking Deb, with patchy dark brown hair, was ready for the nature hike followed by an intimate soak in the hot tub. The tub was surrounded by floppy, purple-headed flowers large enough to hide a hand, a caress, a kiss.

Our next hotel was 15 minutes away at the hot springs in La Fortuna. The springs started higher up and cascaded down the mountain side into containment pools. The highest pool had the hottest water, straight from the base of the volcano. As it flowed downhill it cooled. The lowest pools were just above room temperature but that was still plenty warm enough to remove the thin coating of fake tan I had sprayed onto my skin.

I soaked for as long as I could stand it, wishing the radiation and chemo toxins out of my body. I sweated and drank crystal pure water, then repeated the process. Mud massages made me forget everything but the small powerful hands of the women who turned my flesh into putty. I rinsed in an outdoor grotto in the side of the mountain, swishing the volcanic mud from every part of my body, then emerged slowly, letting the sun warm me. My skin was deliciously soft. Once dry I indulged in the second part of the treatment — the rubbing in of essential oils. I oohed and aahed, never having felt so pampered. It was a moment of mental and emotional well-being that I would wish for anyone dealing with a serious illness.

There was a downside to all that bliss, though.

The next morning, I couldn't stop looking at my feet! They were covered in red blotches that looked ready to blister or bleed at any moment. There were similar lesions on my shoulders and left knee. They looked painful and they were. Sunburns are never fun. The hot springs and mud had chipped away the sunless tanning lotion. I could barely stand to wear a bedsheet or smile. My blistered feet couldn't tolerate the sandal straps. Of course the pavement and sand were too hot to go without shoes, so I didn't travel far.

Man, I had to be careful. I could get cancer. The irony cracked me up. Good thing there was a swim-up bar and beach restaurants with chairs beneath shady palm trees. There *was* a place in heaven for everyone.

For the second week of our trip we rented an apartment in the little town of Samara. It was a quieter, less touristy spot, although every morning we awoke to the croaking of frogs and screeching howler monkeys and exotic birds. Iguana toenails clicked overhead on the tin roof as they skittered upward to bask in the rising sun. We spent three days trying to even out my tan while swimming and walking the beaches in search of sea glass and shells. The undertow, I discovered the hard way, was wicked. I had been standing knee-deep in water one minute. The next, I was tugging my swimsuit bra down from around my head and reaching for my long-gone sunglasses.

The sun was so hot in Costa Rica you had to live in the pool between 1 and 3 p.m., otherwise you fried. This was not a problem at our next and final stop. The all-inclusive resort had a bar with a swim-up side and lots of chilled fruit juices, and I had a big brimmed hat that didn't mind getting wet. We played water volleyball and did aerobics in the water to keep busy. For $20 I received 90 minutes of ecstasy on the beachside massage tables. *All part of the detox regime*, I told myself between moans.

The week went quickly and before we knew it we were cramming everything back into our suitcases. We arrived at our home early in May and slept like we hadn't in three weeks. There really was no place like home. Everything was just how we'd left it and just how we liked it.

My alarm rattled me awake at 5:25 a.m. I leapt to dress for circuit training. I'd been away from it for months and now was the time to get back to it. It felt amazingly good to throw around some weights and run on the treadmill. Sandi and I did our usual abs routine and 20-minute run outside after the class ended. It was a tough grind but I made it through.

After exercising, showering and breakfast, I napped for an hour before racing to make my doctor's appointment with Sandi. She carefully injected me with my third shot of Zoladex and before I could leap off the examination table and stuff my new white shirt into my jeans she was ready with a Band-Aid. She covered the red spot and handed me a spare Band-Aid in case the first one leaked.

"I'll be fine," I told her.

I still haven't got the blood stain out of that shirt either.

I would say things were very back to normal. Or as normal as they would ever be again!

Within a week it was like we'd never been away. Life was like skipping rope; you watched it rise up and down once, twice and then you jumped in. Did I make it? Yes . . . now how to keep jumping?

Everyone wanted to hear that my life was back to normal. I said it was but that wasn't really the truth. I was jumping but life was never going to be the same again. The proof was in the mirror. There was someone else looking back at me. Look at her! Her eyes looked like mine. Same colour . . . a little sadder perhaps and she seemed far older. I was over 50 now, but *she* looked much older than that. Turtle aged, going by the rings around her neck and the stretch marks around her lips.

And her hair! I used to have straight hair that, with the right product and wave of a roller brush and hair dryer, transformed into a gossamer cloud that framed my face with golden highlights. But that poor woman in the mirror had something that looked like black alfalfa sprouts standing straight then swirling right at the top of her head. Curly, fuzzy, poodle-locks. And what colour would you say that was? Dyed-over grey with sun-bleached spiked tips? Wasn't that a Beach Boys style back in the '60s?

It also looked like it would be easy for her to say "Whatever," dive into a big bowl of whipped cream and not surface until her chin doubled and the new scars rested on her belly. So frigging easy to let it all go. Heck, she was old enough. She deserved a break. What did she want to keep fit for?

I turned my head away, not wanting to look anymore. But I did. I took another look at that woman in my mirror. Could that really be me? And if it was, did I need to start changing my perception of myself? Adjust the mental image to match the mess that stood before me? Well, pardon my language, but SCREW THAT! That old lady and me, we were pulling up the bootstraps again and going to Plan B. In fact, we had been on Plan B for three days . . . no meat, dairy, eggs, gluten or sugar. A little veganism for one month to kick-start the flab reversal. One of the side effects of my medication was increased appetite. So be it. I would eat as much as I wanted but it had to be vegetarian. Try gorging on spinach and lentils and see how fat you get. It won't happen. I did spend a large part of the day swinging on the opened fridge door, finding absolutely nothing I wanted before closing it again.

A new wardrobe in larger sizes wasn't for me. I really liked the way I was. The way I was less a bit, a bit that I could manage to lose with some work. It wasn't the first time I'd had to do this. But it was the first time I'd had to talk myself into wanting to do this, and that was the frightening part.

Around the middle of June I realized it had been six months since I'd used any feminine hygiene products. Thanks to the chemo, Zola-dex and tamoxifen I was completely period-free for the first time since my pregnancies almost 30 years ago. This was the moment I had wished for since the very day they started on August 10, 1972. I knew the exact date because my mother did everything but advertise it in the local paper.

There should have been celebration yet for some reason there was a touch of regret in acknowledging the end of something I'd experienced monthly for the major part of my life. I was 13 and a half when I finally learned what all the whispering had been about. I was staying at my friend's cottage when I got that "baseball bat in the stomach" feeling. Some call it butterflies. Mine were more like 50-pound butter turkeys. I hurt from the back of my teeth to my toes. I would get sent home from school, not able to run from the nurse's station to Mom's waiting car without soaking through the two-inch-thick pads. I begged for someone to shoot me, to run me over. It was almost more than my mind could handle. It was disgusting and humiliating. It was gross and obscene and an impediment to my tree climbing and wrestling matches with the guys.

A life sentence for criminals was shorter. Once a month for 39.5 years. That was 474 cycles. Less two pregnancies, so 456. Okay, it also didn't return *right* after my amazing daughter was born, while I breastfed. My amazing son was the result of that. So let's say 450 months. Times seven days for each slot and we were looking at being miserable for 3,150 days out of my life.

Let's not forget the 200 plus Double Fun Days when my dates weren't marked on the calendar and I was caught unprepared. It's not like it was rocket science, but I just somehow refused to give my period the attention it deserved. Even at 50 I forgot and had to bum products from a friend.

And now my periods were gone. If I'd thought of it, I *would* have thrown a farewell party for them. Put all the anti-inflammatory pills, Motrin, tampons, pads, ruined underwear and books on PMS and peri-menopause into a pile out back and had a giant bonfire.

Okay, it's not all roses yet. I'm still getting the cramping, the chocolate bingeing urges and the two days of snapping at my other half. But the odorous inconvenience that made me feel like Carrie soaked in pig blood every single month was finally over. It was farewell to *that* aisle in the drugstore where you always ran into a fellow you hadn't seen in ages seconds after the box of super-cavernous, extra-wide tampons was in hand.

As much as I hated The Curse I had to admit it gave me the greatest two gifts in my life: Karly and Lorne. Periods were something I reviled but understood; something I had to work with so that I could be a woman and a mother. It was an ultimate trade-off. Four hundred and fifty months of painkillers, dark chocolate Lindt bars and zits in exchange for two fascinating lives that I will cherish until I die and then some.

It's not a bad deal when you look at it that way.

I guess the slight melancholy came from understanding I was officially what a friend called "an old spawner." I would never give birth to another human being. *It's a blessing*, I told myself after finding my toothpaste in the fridge. Who would look after me if there was a baby in the house?

16

Grappling Grief Again

I was still swinging on the fridge door trying to find something healthy to eat when the phone rang and my husband answered. It was June 16. I heard him say hello. I heard him say *NO*. I looked up to see his face was crumpled. "No," he said again, but softer.

I remember hearing the fridge buzzing at me to close the door. A horrible dread overwhelmed me.

"Who," I demanded. "*Who?*"

Barry dropped the phone down to his side. "It's your brother," he said. "He's dead."

I can barely write this.

Let's back up.

Two days before, I'd had a call from my sister Kim. She said she had spent an hour trying to talk our brother down off of his garage roof. He had been high in every sense, and suicidal. There was a gathering of ambulance attendants, the police and neighbours.

When Danny visited us in Kelowna earlier in the year he'd left us with a letter. In it he said, "[I] can't predict the future but I know the past hasn't been where I want to spend the rest of eternity. So I'm off to deal with the present. Have given minimal thought to the future, but nothing I've ever planned for has worked out so well anyway!"

On June 14, 2011, my brother, Daniel Robert Harold Saunders, born on March 3, 1957, purposefully jumped from the roof of his garage onto a wooden fence. That wasn't what killed him. After being cleared by the hospital he was arrested under the Mental Health Act. He was judged a danger to himself and spent the night in a jail cell for his own protection. He was returned to the hospital in the morning after complaining about pain. The next day he went into cardiac arrest and died.

We toppled into a whirlpool of confusion. Yes, Danny had been depressed and had a problem with substance abuse. But when we saw him in January he'd said he was happy and clean. Then why had he done this? It made me question what I was doing, why I was trying so hard to stay alive. My life could be considered a mess as well. There was a voice inside that softly asked why I struggled so hard. Wouldn't it be easier just to let it all go, to sink beneath the waves and float away, just like Danny had?

Since birth I'd always followed wherever Danny went — to kindergarten, to school, to western Canada — and this felt the same. The moment I realized it, I also realized I was no longer afraid to die. When there are people waiting for you to join them, the idea of death seems friendlier. You could almost look forward to it.

My grief for my brother turned to anger. I was mad at the entire world, at my brother, at his life, at the hospital, the doctors and the police. I was mad at me for only leaving a message for him to call me back when I knew he was floundering. I wanted to put my fist through a wall. I wanted my body to hurt as much as my soul.

I took it out on people around me. Everything they did was wrong. I snapped at them for breathing. None of it made sense and I didn't feel any better, but I couldn't seem to stop myself, especially when there was a woman inside my mind screaming her head off.

I understand death, how necessary it is in the circle of life. Nobody lasts forever and Danny was with us on borrowed time since a crippling ski accident in his 20s. I tried to be thankful for the years we did have him with us.

A nephew's wife was expecting a child. This was a ray of light. Children were the future. Death was the past. In the end, it wasn't enough to cling to as the waves of sorrow continued crashing on top of my head until under I went again.

Losing someone you love, especially when you feared for your own life, was so messed up. At times like this I had to believe life on earth was hell. It wasn't fair, wasn't easy and not at all the way I thought it should be.

I found some relief in running. Feeling the air coming into my lungs, filling them, exhaling. I was alive and life was good. It was my mother's favourite saying and was on the T-shirts she wore in palliative care. Life is good. I would get over this, move on to the "acceptance" stage of grief, but it was going to be a while yet.

The cheerless pit grew deeper after a friend disclosed her diagnosis of Stage IV pancreatic cancer. It was torturous that I knew only too well what her future held. Another acquaintance, a breast cancer survivor, was trying to deal with a sudden recurrence in the opposite breast after a year on tamoxifen. That was a wake-up slap for me. Wasn't tamoxifen going to be enough to save us? She had another surgery to remove the tumour and was starting chemo. A third friend learned her breast reconstruction would be harder than first thought due to complications from the radiation therapy. It could be done, but with skin grafting and major surgery.

I was glad they phoned to tell me. It's not like I could offer advice but I could be a listener, someone to point out their strengths, to offer help with anything. Being positive without saying everything would be okay. That's how you can help someone battling cancer (although the casseroles and soup are appreciated as well).

Still, each new revelation rattled me. Cancer seemed determined to change everybody's lives . . . patients, family members, friends. What was going on and how did we stop it? I admit I was one of those people who never thought cancer would happen to me. I was too young and being fairly careful. Would that apply to my friends as well? Did they think they were being careful enough?

There are different types of breast cancer tumours. Some have endocrine receptors, meaning they are fed by estrogen or progesterone. Some are labelled HER2, a protein used by cancer cells to grow and multiply. Others are triple negative — unresponsive to estrogen, progesterone, or HER2, and still others can be triple positive.

These classifications provide doctors with valuable information about how the tumour behaves and what treatments may work best. But it all comes down to the same thing, no matter what feeds it. When a cancer starts to turn on and reproduce itself there are some ways you can slow it down.

How do we do that?

By making the inside of our bodies unreceptive to cancer. The bottom line is this: cancer thrives on dehydrated, acidic bodies.

What does that mean?

Our bodies need a balance of acid and alkaline levels, better known as the pH level. Health food stores sell litmus paper to test your levels using urine or saliva. Imbalance and disease can set in when the body is dealing with too much stress and acid-forming foods. That's your refined sugar, processed foods, red meat, alcohol, pop, and foods made with white flour.

What keeps you alkaline? Green vegetables, fresh fruits, whole grains and, believe it or not, something super simple — the juice of half a fresh lemon or one tablespoon of lemon juice in warm water every day. Lemon juice is acidic but converts to an alkaline, or basic, residue when metabolized by the body. Easy. Add a sensible diet, lots of water and sleep, regular exercise and you're good to go for the day! Possibly for the rest of your long, disease-free life.

Dr. Robert Young has a book you might be interested in called *The pH Miracle*. In it he stresses the importance of maintaining a balance and even says it will promote weight loss, increase stamina and more importantly . . . it gives you a stronger immune system. And that's what we need. More armour if a cancer ever starts. Keeping a growth small gives the immune system and the medical profession a better chance of eliminating it. But you have to do your part.

Are you taking a multivitamin daily to ensure you're getting everything you need? How about antioxidants like blueberries and broccoli? Vitamin D — getting enough of that every day? Are you exercising four times a week for at least 20 minutes each time? Remember that cancer cells hate oxygen so the more you breathe in deeply, the better the knock-out punch. Excess weight leads to increased levels of estrogen, which increases the risk of developing breast cancer.

Are you waiting to get thirsty before you drink something? That means you are already dehydrated. Are you drinking sugarless and aspartame-free fluids? Are you eating organic or at least washing off all your fruits and veggies with a teaspoon of vinegar or hydrogen peroxide and a cup of water before cutting or consuming them?

Having said all that, I have to admit life with a side order of tamoxifen and Zoladex was not a picnic. Tamoxifen worked by blocking the effects of estrogen in breast tissue while Zoladex stopped the ovaries from making estrogen. But there was a price to pay. Any willpower I'd had was shredded. I know I'd vowed to eat sensibly but these drugs kidnapped me. I stuffed my pie hole with as many fattening things as I could find despite knowing what it would do to my cholesterol readings, to my waistline, to my guilty conscience. On one occasion I managed to eat an entire bucket of greasy chicken. Neither the act nor any of the chicken was shared with Barry. It was a shameful moment. And I won't even mention how much wine I was drinking.

The bingeing didn't make me feel any better, but I couldn't seem to stop. Even if my hands had been tied behind my back I would have shoved my head into the box of Cocoa Puffs. It was pathetic. There was no control. No staying power.

Whatever was in the Zoladex and tamoxifen had me trampolining on highs and lows like an Olympic gymnast. I could go from joy to manic depression in the time it took to check my watch. There wasn't enough food in the fridge to satisfy me. I became defeated as my waist spilled over the top of my pants, the buttons on my blouses bowed and the number on the bathroom scale soared like a free bird.

I couldn't sleep, lost almost all interest in sex, and the hot flashes came faster than traffic light changes. I put clothes on, I took clothes off. This took up a good portion of my day. How did women work while on this stuff? Who had time to accomplish anything? I had Japanese hand fans by each phone and work desk, in each vehicle and my purse. I packed spare shirts in the car and kept mini handwipes and deodorant nearby at all times. At least that issue was manageable and the wipes were very handy on fried chicken days. I used to get embarrassed fanning myself at a restaurant after eating a hot pepper or after Barry commenting, "You take handfuls of antioxidant capsules and now you order fries with gravy?"

And then I happened to look in a mirror again.

When would I learn?

No, not another nose growing. Not longer lashes, but you are thinking along the right lines. I was looking at more hair but it wasn't growing on top of my head. Thanks to the hormone suppression, I now had a beard.

"This is silly," I told myself, "I can fix this. It's not the end of the world."

A girlfriend used facial wax so I bought some. You heat it up, apply and pull off. Simple. The obnoxious burnt wax fumes lasted three days in our kitchen and a week inside the microwave. Seems I overheated it. Ignoring this, I spread the molten wax on my jaw line with a flat stick and let it harden as recommended. After hopping around in pain for three minutes, I had to peel the wax back. Holy Mother! It felt like my face was coming off with each tug. Tears welled up and my body went into one long hot flash. Then Barry came home to find me struggling to pull my sweater over my head. "What the heck is that smell? Was that dinner?" he asked, sounding mortified.

I left the sweater over my head and ran for the truck. "I'll be back in a minute, honey."

Crap.

Once in the truck I pulled the sweater back down, grabbed a bandana from the glove box and tied it across the bottom half of my face, bandit style. I headed for Carolyn's salon at the mall. The receptionist's scream echoed across the far parking lot. She thought I had come to rob them.

"Help me get this wax off my face or someone might get hurt," I told her.

The young woman bolted for help.

Carolyn fixed me up, but it took some doing and some colourful words from both of us, especially after I smacked her hand away once. A plethora of rainbows drifted out of the esthetics room before we were done. Besides the residual pain, I was left with swollen cheeks and new creases along my jaw. It attracted lots of attention to the beard.

As usual, I had learned the hard way.

17

The Troops Rally

The beginning of August marked the end of my first year as a breast cancer statistic. I was trying to get back to normal, but it wasn't coming easy. I was starting to think maybe I'd never reach the ease and scope of my pre-cancer physical activities. I never realized what I could do before. What I had.

Maybe the process seemed long because it takes awhile to go through the stages of grief. There are five of them — denial (Surface Girl, thinking I was only going to be mildly inconvenienced by this cancer), anger (why me?), bartering (I'll be a good girl if you only let me live through this), depression (life is crap) and acceptance (let's learn to work with what we have). Unfortunately, almost no one progresses in an orderly way through the stages. There's a lot of to-and-fro-ing, gaining ground and then seemingly losing it.

Before I started acting more responsibly, I had to go through all those stages. I was a defensive, some days waffling, wannabe commercial for cancer prevention. It was in my heart at least. One day I would be Deb the warrior queen brandishing my anti-cancer sword in the air. The next day I would drop it on my head.

Who was I kidding? How much more of this goody-two-shoes routine could I take? When I quit smoking I told myself I would only quit for a bit. For one year and then I could go back to smoking. My mind bought the lie and before I knew it a year had passed. The last thing I wanted to do then was smoke a cigarette and go through the agony of quitting again.

Maybe that strategy would work? Just one year on this new anti-cancer regime. After that . . . well, hopefully it would stick and I could do it without thinking about it.

It's such a cat and mouse game. I waged a war with cancer and for now I'm the victor. But there could be cells inside of me, dormant now thanks to the tamoxifen and Zoladex, waiting for me to slip back to the old me, the chocolate-gorging, wine-swilling exercise wanker (with beautiful long hair). If I didn't change what gave me cancer in the first place, and no one will say exactly what that was, then it could happen again. It was only a matter of time. And how much of that did I have? Enough to have a grandchild conceived, born and fast-forwarded to their high school graduation? The mere thought of having to hold my breath for that long worried me. Wait a minute. Worrying caused stress which . . .

See? I was doomed! I was barely holding myself above water, my nose already tilted to the sky so I could breathe. There was a depth of despair out there I had never been to and hoped never to get to. How many wishes was my mom going to grant me?

I often wondered where my line was. At what point would it be too much? I'd tried all my childhood to catch up to my brother, but he was always faster, stronger, smarter. In the end, he had chosen a destructive path, and I worried I might follow him again. Could I come through all of this in one piece or would it get me too?

After Danny died, I fell into a black abyss for two solid weeks. It was hard to find the energy to do anything, to find a reason to keep going. I ate a lot of comfort food. With the anti-cancer drugs driving my hunger to a new high, it was easy to pack on an extra 10 pounds. There was *always* something unpleasant to deal with.

My lung capacity was still not where I felt it should be. I was five months post-treatments. Sandi and I still jogged 40 minutes two to three times a week, but at the end of the run, if I exerted myself, I couldn't seem to catch a breath. More than once I ended up struggling to get air, tears of frustration welling in my bugged-out eyes. The more I tried, the more frustrated I got, which upset me further, clamping a band around my airway. Sandi reminded me to exhale as much as I could before trying to inhale. It took a few seconds to catch up. A few terrifying seconds before it passed.

Breathe in. Breathe out. Don't cry, don't cry, that would make it worse.

I was usually bent double with my hands on my knees before the gasping eased. Sandi suggested I might want to get the shortness of breath checked out, and before the month passed we were off to Prince George to see a heart specialist.

His report stated my "ejection fraction," or the percentage of blood in the left ventricle of my heart that actually got pumped to my body, including my lungs, had been reduced by 5 to 10 percent. When I exerted myself my left ventricle muscle didn't have the snap needed to deliver as much oxygen-rich blood as required. I got dizzy, couldn't catch my breath and gasped for air. The cardiologist said this could possibly repair itself.

Probable cause — pushing myself too flipping hard throughout the chemo. *Look at me! I can still jog and swim and hike and bike. Cancer won't slow me down. No, it can't catch me. Run, Deb, RUN!*

Treatment — more pills, this time to slow my heart down a notch, another to lower my cholesterol level. Your heart might repair itself. It might not. Take one baby aspirin and don't call me in the morning. Next . . .

We returned to Houston even more deflated than usual. Where was bottom on this downslide?

Relying solely on medical system personnel to look after your overall health is not recommended anymore. They have become unreasonably busy and your annual checkups could slip through the cracks. You have to learn to be your own best advocate. You have to make sure your physician is following through on a valid concern. Sometimes they take the "wait even longer and we'll see . . ." attitude. Sometimes that is not in your best interest.

I've had doctors make me feel useless. One burnt the inside of my thigh with a lamp during an internal exam. He told me I had herpes, sounding disgusted as he said it. It turned out, after he almost ended my marriage with that announcement, that it was a tear from a tampon insertion gone wrong. It took months to heal because of its location in such a moist area. But it did heal and I did not have genital herpes. I also did not have that doctor anymore.

After experiencing the TIAs from the Ritalin, I was very leery of taking any meds. That was a joke, given that tamoxifen increased the risk of uterine cancer. But what was the alternative? If I stopped the daily dosage and had a recurrence, I would kick myself for the rest of my days. If I kept taking it and ended up with liver or uterine cancer, I would kick myself for the rest of my days.

It was a no-win situation.

But I was alive and still able to do most of what I did one year ago. I also had a new respect for good health, for being able to do something without hurting. I had taken it for granted all of those years.

As if it were a bonus for finally "getting it," Mom once again worked her magic. There was to be a 10-year reunion, a welcome event with girlfriends I'd met in the '90s. Back then all of us were new to Houston, strangers, eager to meet other interesting women in town. Someone to lunch with, to swap stories with, you know how that goes. We began calling it our One Hour Lunch Club and invited other women to join. Before long there were a dozen of us. We had to book reservations, something unheard of in this town, so we could sit together. We talked about food and health, but better yet, about feelings, relationships and sex. "No holds barred" was the motto.

Without knowing it, we had become a strong support group for one another.

Then they started to move away. One by one they left for warmer places, back to South Africa, one home to New Zealand, one 12 hours south to Nakusp, and on and on. Only Sandi and I were left behind.

This particular year my mother managed to align the stars so that the Kiwi was coming to Canada for a visit right when I needed to see her the most. The South African was in Vancouver and flew north to meet us. Sandi and I gathered a posse of good women at my home and had the harmonica, guitars and singsong going until the wee-est of hours. Buoyed by so much love, I wanted to be there for them as much as they were there for me.

Their visit rekindled my anti-cancer crusade. I mean, what if any of these women I loved was forced to travel the road I'd been on for the past year? Who would be there for them, for women I'd yet to meet?

For three glorious days I thrived on and reveled in the laughter and the reminiscing, the good times we had and were making. Then, sadly, we parted, the bubble of love floating me along for another week. *I am valued for who I am. I am strong. I'm alive.*

Repeat as often as necessary.

As I've said, with ADD you don't often experience the highs without the lows. The crash always came and even after 51 years I never saw it coming. It crept up slowly. It was harder to get up in the mornings. I couldn't think of anything important enough to rise and shine for. Sure, my blog and writing waited. My search for the healthiest recipes. The kids and their lives. Our friends and their lives. But somehow, it wasn't enough.

I slept and slept and when I awoke, I felt drained. More tired and sad than I can ever remember feeling. It wasn't so much melancholy as it was a vacuum of nothingness. Like the sunshine had been sucked out of my soul. My down days had never lasted this long before.

I think I was feeling abandoned. First my brother, then some friends claimed by cancer and now by people that I loved. I had been surrounded by their good wishes and joy for life and now it was gone. I wasn't sure I could deal with it all. I had held their hands and then had to let go of the warmth and the support. The party hats and crutches had been stowed. It was time to stand on my own, but it wasn't happening. I was face down in the gutter and finding it hard to breathe. Barry tried to console me but it wasn't enough to reverse my sense of loss, not just of my brother and friends but of my past life, everything that used to make sense.

For three days I stayed in bed or on the couch until minutes before Barry came home from the pharmacy. Then I'd drag myself into the kitchen to open a tin of this or a bag of that, food I neither cared about nor wanted. Afterwards I would return to the bed or the couch or pretend to work at the computer.

One morning I put on my housecoat, shuffled down the stairs to our office and sat before my computer's blank screen. I was determined to blog about this. I had been honest about everything else, had shared every pain and annoyance and embarrassing moment up to then. This blackness needed to be recorded as well.

It took a few moments of typing about nothing and then it began to come. The words of pain, the anger, the disappointment, the feelings of loss and disruption and sorrow. I moved onto a list of everything I had been through and what I was still dealing with. The list grew and grew until I sat in a hole deeper than I could ever hope to manage. I couldn't do it.

All I *could* do was cry and sob some more. And more. And then I heard something. Was that my brother calling me? I looked around, straining my ears. Did Danny want me where he was? Was he asking me to come?

A voice inside of me asked, *Wouldn't you love to be there with*

him and Mom? Wouldn't you just love to rest for a while, to be quiet?
To stop hurting?

For the first time in three days I began to feel relief. Maybe it
could be that simple. Why did I have to make everything in my
life so hard? I had spent years swimming upstream. It was time to
stop swimming. Time to let go and float downstream. I could feel
the relief simply having made the decision.

A picture came into my head. I saw Barry's hunting guns lined
up in a locked cupboard in the next room. And I knew where the
key was, where the bullets were. And I knew it was something else
that I *could* do.

That last idea made me cry even harder until something in my
mind told me I had to get myself out of that chair. My fingers were
dead. They had nothing more to type. I got up and walked toward
the doorway. I was at a crossroads. Ten steps ahead to that room.
Or . . .

I had no thoughts as my feet made the decision, carrying me
upstairs and away faster than I had moved in days. Tears and snot
and hair stuck to my face and my vision was blurred. I yanked the
phone drawer open, grabbed my address book and found Sandi's
cell phone number. Dialing, praying, hoping, please be there. I've
never needed anybody so bad, so now!

And she answered the phone. She was working in Emergency and
I said, "Sandi, I need help. I can't stop crying and I think I'm suicidal."

"Come in," she told me. "Get a friend to drive you. Call Dorothy."

I didn't bother to get dressed. I grabbed my purse and jumped
into the Suburban, trying not to think about anything. Still, the
sobbing kept renewing itself. I drove the one block to my friend's
home. Dorothy and Henry were working on their lawn. One look
at me and Dorothy dropped her rake and came running.

"What happened? Are you okay?"

My body shook as the tears ran. "I need to go to the hospital.
Can you drive me?"

I was enfolded in Dorothy's embrace as Henry ran to grab her purse. We were on the road within minutes. We cried the whole way to Smithers as I told her everything. How I had only meant to write down the poison inside of me, how it had turned into a nightmare that I was still in the middle of. That I didn't want to live anymore. And I meant it.

Sandi met us in the ER although she had another physician check me in as, she explained, it was all too close to her. I was given an Ativan, an anti-anxiety drug, and Dorothy left to buy us a latte as backup.

I spent the afternoon sitting on the edge of a hospital bed, completely drained and dazed. What had happened? And how did I get back to me from here?

Barry arrived after work, rattled to the core. He brought flowers. I was happy to see him and silently shook in his arms. I now felt guilty, embarrassed and sorry for the trouble I was causing. The Ativan had staunched the tears but the heaviness on my shoulders was worse than ever. I hated being in hospital. I worried someone might see me, might know that I had dropped the stoic ball, had confessed to needing help. How could I set an example of how to fight cancer when I had crumbled beneath it all?

A mental health professional came to my room. He handed me a sheet of paper and asked that I write about what had triggered my sadness. I was also to write down the names and numbers of people I could call if these feelings of destruction came again. I was to carry that paper with me at all times. I kept nodding my head at the man. He recommended antidepressants. I never heard most of what he said. Something about follow-up appointments in Houston or blah, blah. I just wanted to go home and crawl back into bed.

I got to do that the following morning. I said I felt better although I felt nothing still. Numb and dark. I received more Ativan to keep my eyes dry, my head empty. I would deal with all of this another day.

———

I'm happy to say the antidepressants eventually did their work and the clouds did clear. I slowly climbed out of the hole and resumed my weary battle to survive. The "out the other end" champagne had been consumed but I wondered if maybe I'd jumped the gun with the bubbly. I had finished the treatments but I had to log five years cancer-free before I could declare "I made it!" If, that was, I *did* make it.

I had yet to find out if indeed we did get it all or if there was some little piece that survived, starting to multiply someplace else as we speak. I didn't know what to trust anymore. My body and then my mind had let me down once. Would they do it again?

One-third of women with hormone-dependent tumours (like mine) will have a recurrence and in more than half of those it will happen within five years after surgery. Because I opted for the adjunct therapy (the chemo and radiation) combined with surgery, my chance of a recurrence goes way down. I think I'm at a 3–5 percent chance. It's still enough to make you worry. I've been beaten by better odds.

Saying you're a survivor implies the war is over, but for me the battle had just begun. This was going to be a life-long journey of learning and doing what I could to survive. I needed to find the determination to keep the numbers on my side. It was a betting game with no guarantees and I had to do what I could to help myself. If that meant swallowing large fish oil and green tea capsules (antioxidants), stuffing in the blueberries by the handful, drinking the green spirulina algae with my nose pinched, dragging my butt to the swimming pool, drinking water not wine, filling my lungs with fresh air, then that was what I would do. I would try to keep fighting because, as Mom loved to say, "Life is good." It's also for the living, so I was either in or I was out. Guess I needed that break from myself and my grief because the urge to kill cancer before it killed me had returned.

Possibly, when I was on my last breath, when I had lived a much longer life, I would finally declare myself a bona-fide breast cancer survivor and not merely a wannabe. Until that happened, look out cancer. It was Game On!

On February 18, 2012, it was time to celebrate again. It had been a year since my last dose of radiation and I was feeling wise beyond my years, almost euphoric, angelic, eager to help others in any way needed. I notice and care for others more, share more, bake more, ignore the house and write more. I am ready to tell the world about my trip down this bumpy road and give others confidence that they too can deal with it.

I am also still on antidepressants. Saying that is hard for me. I went so long with my head above water all on my own. I looked cancer in its ugly face and didn't run. I held my ground and fought back. But . . . sometimes it got the best of me.

Realizing I needed help was the biggest and most important step. Now I can stay in the sunshine and keep the dark clouds at bay. I removed the pictures of my mother and brother from my dresser but I'll put them back one day . . . when I know I'm ready. I'm not the type to postpone hardship or rely on a crutch, but I was harder on myself than any person should be. I've stopped doing that. I'm learning yoga . . . slow . . . smooth . . . gentle.

Maybe part of the well-being I feel is chemically induced but trying to get there on my own wasn't the answer either. My head is clear and my thoughts are positive. I sometimes cry for my losses but I can stop when I want to. I can get out of bed when I want. I can tell my husband how much I love and appreciate him and mean it.

Bottom line . . . it's all in how you look at things. It's all about attitude. I'm still here, still kicking and ready to make a difference in the world for somebody else. I have worked hard to finish this book, the possibility of a recurrence working like a flame beneath my butt. I get up and get moving. Time could be short; then again time could go on. I'll take whatever I can get.

I believe all things happen to us for a reason. I was meant to go down that road, and my friends and family were meant to be there with me. Thank you to everyone for every little or large action you took, whether it was merely a smile or a kind word, a little surprise or a house to borrow.

I urge everyone reading this to take a good, hard look at your lifestyle. At your dietary choices. At your stress levels. Be honest and be prepared to be surprised. It's going to take more than a tablespoon of ground flax seed on your oatmeal every morning but with time and knowledge you too can stop running and learn to stand up to cancer.

To your battle stations, everyone. Ready, aim . . .

Appendix A

Weapons to Arm Yourself With

I once asked Barry's 95-year-young grandma what her secret to long life was. Alice said, "I grow my own vegetables, eat lots of fruit and fish, I walk every day and I have a little nip now and again." She added the last touch with a wink.

Here are TEN weapons to arm you in your fight against cancer. Whether it runs in your family or not, whether you feel fine or have been recently diagnosed, NOW is the time to start changing things so we can get those rising numbers of cancer victims reversed. Be brave and start kicking cancer right where it deserves. Start today and possibly, with a bit of hope, we can slow down this forest fire or stamp it out all together (double meaning intended).

1   QUIT SMOKING. Yes, you can do it. The secret? Just stop. Chew gum, put on a patch, sleep for three days straight, do whatever you can to get through. It will be rough, especially the first day, but every breath after that gets easier and cleaner. Make sure your last puff was just that because even one puff years later can make you have to go through the entire thing again. Once you become a non-smoker, from the first second onward, you have to

tell yourself that is what you are and never, ever change your mind.

2 PUT BETTER WEAPONS INSIDE YOUR BODY. Drop the empty calories of white breads for whole grains and brown rice products. Pump up the organic or carefully washed fruits and vegetables and eat less red meat and animal fats. Take a supplement of 1–2000 milligram of vitamin D and eat leafy green vegetables, berries and nuts. And yes, ground flax seed.

3 AVOID SUGAR. Sugar is another enemy. Besides causing excess weight gain, it feeds cancer cells. It's like buying your enemy bullets to kill you with. I'm not saying to never have a bowl of ice cream or a donut again. I'm saying to cut it way back. And use natural sweeteners like dates, figs, honey, maple syrup or palm sugars whenever possible. Start a treat day — a time to spoil yourself after resisting all week. Think before you eat or drink anything. Will this help my body or weaken it?

4 DRINK LESS ALCOHOL. Way less. The connection between alcohol and cancer is astounding. Recommendations straight from the Canadian Cancer Society are less than one drink a day for women and up to two for men. No stockpiling for the weekend! There is no recommended safe level if you've had cancer.

5 EXERCISE EVERY DAY. Oxygen kills cancer cells, but we're not getting enough. We need to get up and get going. Take yoga, tai chi, a gym class, walking, cycling, hiking.

Just get off that couch more often than not. Maintain a healthy body weight because obesity is a contributing factor to cancer.

6 DRINK GOOD WATER and lots of it. Being made up of 50–75 percent water, your body depends on you replenishing it hourly to do all that it has to do, including flush nasty toxins from your system. Ozonized, natural spring, artesian or mineral waters are the healthiest. Stripping all the minerals from water is not the answer, which happens when using most common filter systems, distilled, reverse osmosis, or de-ionized water.

7 SEE YOUR DOCTOR for regular checkups. Don't put off having that lump in your breast or the pain in your stomach or back looked at by a professional. Find out your personal health history from your relatives; start asking and documenting. Pass that valuable information on to your doctor. It could save your life!

8 GET INFORMED on other ways to boost your immune system. It's the best weapon you have for fighting cancer. Buy books and magazines, watch health shows on television. Search out healthy recipes and share them with friends.

9 DONATE. Every volunteer hour, every penny raised, gets a cancer victim one step closer to putting the disease behind them. My mini metastasis would not have been detected as early as one year ago. Your support makes it all possible and, as a former cancer patient, I can't thank you enough.

10 Spread the word and then practise what you preach. Tell everyone you know how they can fight cancer. It may be hard at first, but once you figure out substitutes for your weaknesses, like buying baked brown rice crackers instead of potato chips, it will get easier. Better yet, make Kale Chips; the recipe is included in this book.

It's never too early to start fighting for your life.

Appendix B

Favourite Recipes

My cupboard is crowded with a multitude of recipe books. I have folders to keep copies of the recipes we like so I can use them again. They are labeled under headings like fish, chicken, vegetables, sauces, etc. Most are your basic recipes that call for things I can change to a healthier option. I usually switch any butter or oils called for to coconut oil (the kind for baking without the coconut smell or taste). I substitute egg whites for whole eggs, use brown rice flour instead of any flour (I experiment with different flours for baked goods) and use only natural sweeteners. It's amazing how many recipes you can use pureed dates for instead of a cup or two of sugars. The salt I use is ground dulse (seaweed) powder or sea salt and half of what is called for. We abide by the Canada Food Guide rule, "one half of your plate is filled with vegetables, one quarter protein or alternative and one quarter with grain products." We avoid white rice, white pasta and white potatoes in favour of brown rice, brown rice pastas and baked yams.

With a bit of effort and research, you can turn your meals into great works of natural goodness. And fight cancer at the same time.

On my web site at www.debilynsmith.com I have a section for recipes. The list is growing all the time and I encourage you to send some of your favourite healthy recipes, with a picture, for me to post.

Although some of the recipes are from my former days of high fat and "anything goes," there are also very healthy options that I use as often as I can. Mostly to curb that dreaded sweet tooth or snack craving. These include my three favourites: Halibut Stir-Fry, Sinless Chocolate Macaroons and Anti-Cancer Kale Chips, which I copy here for you.

Halibut Stir-Fry

Being so close to the coast affords us a freezer full of halibut, but you are welcome to use any firm, white fish. This is the most colourful low-calorie recipe I have ever made. It is quite flexible for vegetable choices and is so filling you can skip the rice or noodles.

Ingredients

1 TBSP brown rice flour
⅓ cup low-sodium chicken or vegetable stock (note: need 1 cup stock altogether)
1 TBSP lemon juice
½ tsp dried oregano
½ tsp honey
¼ tsp lemon pepper
⅔ cup chicken or vegetable stock
1 cup thinly sliced carrot
1 cup diced butternut (or other) squash
1 cup broccoli or cauliflower florets
⅔ cup frozen peas
1 TBSP cooking oil (olive or coconut is the best for you)
1¼–2 pounds de-boned halibut (cut into ¾ inch cubes)
2 green onions sliced

Instructions

Sauce: Combine the first six sauce ingredients in a small bowl and set aside. Heat the ⅔ cup amount of stock in a non-stick wok or frying pan on medium-high heat. Add carrot, squash and florets. Cook uncovered, stirring occasionally, until tender crisp (about five minutes), then add peas. Heat and stir two minutes. Turn into a medium-size bowl. Wipe out wok.

Reheat wok on medium-high until hot. Add oil and halibut. Stir-fry until opaque (two minutes). Stir the rice flour sauce before adding to the halibut. Heat and stir another minute until boiling and thickened. Add vegetables and the green onions. Stir until heated through. Makes about five cups. Enjoy!

Sinless Chocolate Macaroons

These cookies have literally ended my chocolate bar cravings. I always keep some on hand. A snap to prepare and the kids love them.

Ingredients
2 cups unsweetened medium shredded coconut
½ cup sifted cocoa powder
½ cup pitted dates chopped fine
¼ cup water
2 eggs (or use equivalent of egg white)
2 tsp pure vanilla extract
1 TBSP finely ground flax seed or flax mixture called Nutra-Cleanse

Instructions
Preheat oven to 350°F and line a baking sheet with parchment paper.

In a saucepan over medium-low heat, stir the chopped dates with the water and keep stirring until a chunky "honey" consistency, about 8 minutes. Add more water if necessary. Cool for 10 minutes.

In a bowl, place the coconut, vanilla, cocoa, flax seeds and eggs. Add cooled dates and mix well.

Using your fingers pat ¼ cup or less into a flat cookie and place on the prepared pan. Bake for 14–18 minutes until firmish. Once they harden a bit, they become nice and chewy. Note: I have also baked them in a greased square pan and cut into bars.

Vegan: substitute eggs with 2 TBSP finely ground flax seed mixed with 6 TBSP water.

Anti-Cancer Kale Chips

Making kale chips is one of the easiest ways to get more greens into your family. This proven antioxidant boosts your immune system, giving you the tools to combat cancer. Make plenty as they will go fast once everyone catches on to how amazing they are!

(Thanks to Carlie for bringing these to my attention!)

Ingredients

Kale stems nice and full, washed and patted dry
Sea salt or Mrs. Dash
Olive oil cooking spray

Instructions

Remove the stalky stem of the kale as much as possible by sliding your hand down the centre and pulling the leafy part away from the stem. Discard the stems or put them aside to make vegetable broth with other veggies.

Tear the larger kale pieces into silver dollar-size bits. Place them on a cookie sheet, giving them space to dry as they cook. Do not heap them on top of each other.

Spray very lightly with olive oil cooking spray. Gingerly sprinkle sea salt or Mrs. Dash across them.

Pop into a preheated oven of 300°F, turning the temperature down to 250°F immediately. Leave the oven door open a small inch if possible to help the steam escape.

Check every 10 minutes for dryness. When completely dry, after about 30 minutes, remove and cool before serving. Place any remaining chips in a tight sealing glass or tin container. Use in the next day or two to ensure crispness.

Leftover Quinoa Fried "Rice"

There is no rice in this recipe, but the quinoa comes out tasting just as good or better than if you had used rice. This is the healthier option and one that is handy for leftover quinoa.

Ingredients

3 cups or any significant amount of leftover quinoa cooked and chilled

3 TBSP olive or coconut oil divided

2 eggs or egg whites beaten with a fork

1 TBSP water

1 onion minced

1 garlic clove minced

2 stalks celery diced small

Other veggies you have, like zucchini, carrot, green or red peppers diced fine (optional)

Leftover meat diced (optional)

¼ cup frozen peas

1 TBSP soy sauce

Chopped fresh cilantro (optional)

Instructions

This is made like your favourite fried rice recipe, or use mine:

Mix the eggs with the water. Heat ½ TBSP of oil in a small skillet and cook the egg without stirring. Flip once. Remove from heat and place the egg on a cutting board and shred or slice into thin short strips. Set aside.

In a wok or large frying pan with sides, heat the remaining oil. Add the onion, garlic, celery and optional veggies and stir-fry until they are soft. Add any leftover meat. Heat through.

Add the chilled quinoa and frozen peas. Keep stirring until the quinoa is heated through, adding a TBSP or two of water if it sticks to the pan. Sprinkle with fried egg, soy sauce and optional cilantro. Serve!

Mediterranean Dip

This recipe came from a good friend, a trained chef, in Kamloops, B.C. Barb's recipe is as easy as she promised.

Ingredients
    2 red peppers, seeded and chopped
    1 eggplant, chopped, skin on
    1 purple/red onion chopped
    1 entire head of garlic, peeled and chopped
    2 TBSP extra virgin olive oil
    Salt and pepper

Instructions
Preheat oven to 450°F. Chop all veggies (into fairly large chunks preferably) and put into a Dutch oven or wide pan. Drizzle the olive oil over all the veggies and put into the oven. Stir well after 20 minutes. After 45 minutes total, take out of oven and let cool. Put into a food processor and pulse for 10 seconds until smooth but chunky. Serve with a very firm cracker. Enjoy!

Salmon Noodle Bowl

Another excellent anti-cancer dish that is fast and possibly uses a few straggling ingredients in your cupboards. Full of antioxidants like salmon, spinach, carrots, ginger and onion. Excellent choice!

Ingredients

4 cups vegetable or low-sodium chicken broth (preferably homemade)

2 TBSP teriyaki sauce

1 carrot peeled and cut in thin rings

⅛ cup fresh ginger julienned or chopped

6–8 ounces of skinless, boneless raw salmon cut into small bite-size pieces

Rice, pea or shrimp noodles

1 cup fresh spinach shredded or cut into bite-size pieces

1 green onion sliced

Instructions

Heat the stock with the carrot and ginger in it. Cook until the vegetables are tender. Add the rest of the ingredients except the green onions and cook over medium heat five minutes until done. Sprinkle with the green onions and serve!

You can add raw egg, sesame seeds or other veggies.

Appendix C

Returning the Favour

It's not uncommon to feel an overwhelming desire to give back, or to help with the whole cancer situation in any way possible once you've repaired from your own issues.

I recently had a very informative chat with a woman named Maria at the Canadian Cancer Society. I called their toll-free number because it had been given to me when I first learned I had breast cancer in case I wanted to be paired with a breast cancer survivor. I vaguely remember being told about it, amidst a thousand other things more important to remember at the time. You initially get hit with such a barrage of info sheets, booklets and pamphlets on top of your own research through the Internet and books. At one time I had seven books about cancer stacked beside my bed for some gruesome late-night reading.

Sadly, I forgot all about it until I was rooting through my "cancer bag" information sheets and there it was.

I called them now that my treatments had finished because I was going to add their information to my book and wanted to make sure the service was still available. And, I admit, I was curious about what I had missed out on.

The CCS has a pool of volunteers who are cancer survivors. These generous people are willing to be contacted by cancer patients and their families in need of a mentor or friend to help them down the new path they've suddenly found themselves on. These volunteers have been there and are now trained to help you. They take courses on how to better relate what they went through so that you will benefit the most from their knowledge. For better or for worse, you have someone willing to help you understand what you will be facing.

Where was my head at when I was given the number? I sure could have used this service!

I think the majority of my high anxiety throughout the entire ordeal was from never knowing what exactly I faced next. The cancer books and info pamphlets told me basically what was going to happen, but they never quite got to the real truths of everything. Like, are their hair dryers in the hospital rooms? Don't laugh — it was the difference between packing an overnight suitcase or an overnight bag for my two-day hospital stay. I never travel light. I hate needing something that I have at home, so I drag everything with me.

Of course I had plenty of serious questions. Like what happens after the biopsy comes back positive? What happens after surgery? What is this staging everyone talks about? Are you put on a special diet? Questions like what does the chemo drug feel like when it hits your veins? Does it burn or sting? (No, it doesn't.) Can I wear nail polish when going through chemotherapy? (You can, but preferably you shouldn't in case something goes really sideways.) How big will the incisions be for a second surgery? Will they use the same scars? How long will I be on a couch after surgery? Will I be able to do much the first few days?

I was so impressed with the program that I got thinking, *There's a list of things I would like to share with the people coming behind me, as well.* That's why I am recording it all in a book.

Marie told me that one year after my last treatment, I am eligible to sign up as a CCS volunteer. I filled out an application and got a reply back about the next steps. If accepted, there will be online interviews, orientation and training. Phone calls exchanged. It sounded like a very thorough process. Psychological training and counselling included. This will be a person who seriously wants to help you. The old "pay it forward." Do for others what others have done for you, possibly? Whatever their reasons, these people are available.

Man, I could have used some of that help; someone to say, "Whoa. Relax. It's all going to be okay no matter what happens. Quit suffering. It doesn't have to be this way."

If you are a survivor of any type of cancer and want to volunteer, or if you are going through the cancer trip and want a peer to talk to, please, please call 1-888-939-3333 right now.

There are many ways to give back to the CCS. Fundraisers ensure the research to deter or end cancer keeps progressing. Like the Relay for Life held across Canada every June. Run or Walk for the Cure with CIBC or in a marathon like the Terry Fox Run. Help sell daffodils every spring or do what you can to keep the money coming. Every bit does count. I'm a prime example, as one year ago my micro metastasis in my lymph node would not have been found. I have all the people that gave to the CCS to thank for that.

Your time can be as valuable as your cash. Programs like Look Good Feel Better (LGFB) need people to lift spirits. The LGFB program brings female cancer patients together for a few hours of applying free makeup samples from an impressive list of donors. We were taught how to draw in missing eyebrows and lip lines. How to care for and wear a wig. How to apply concealer to the dark circles beneath our eyes. It was a day never to forget, especially during a hot flash when the strangers on either side of me turned and instinctively began to blow cold air on me.

Hospitals and clinics need volunteers to push coffee and book carts. There is a list of ways you can help just by contacting your nearest provincial CCS.

It always feels better to give than to receive.

Appendix D

Recommended Reading

I have read many books on cancer since all this started. In the beginning I bought the *Intelligent Patient Guide to Breast Cancer*, a book sometimes handed out to new breast cancer patients. I used it like a bible to see what was coming next in the chain of events. (Actually, less like a bible and more like a Stephen King novel.) It's pretty close to the truth and I would highly recommend you buy one or go to your local cancer clinic and ask for one. The clinics usually have their own libraries you can borrow a plethora of information from.

Helping to fine-tune my life from a diet perspective, my intuitive stepdaughter Lindsay sent me a stack of books for Christmas. On the top was David Wolfe's *Superfoods*, which really opened my eyes. David claims it's possible at any age to change our destiny into one of pain-free, vibrant health using the power of these so-called superfoods. These include acai and goji berries, cacao, coconut, spirulina, AFA blue-green algae among others. He states that these foods are known to reduce the severity and improve the symptoms of all types of cancers and other diseases.

For now, I think I'll try to eat healthy from what I can find at my local supermarket. There isn't an organic section, but I can find the odd bag of organic gala apples or box of blueberries when I read labels. The rest, I buy as is and wash before using in a mixture of vinegar or hydrogen peroxide and water: Add ¼ cup 3% H_2O_2 to a sink full of cold water. Soak light vegetables (lettuce, etc.) 20 minutes, thicker skinned vegetables (like cucumbers) for 30 minutes. Drain and dry. This will help them to stay fresh longer.

I check for low or no sugar, starch, fat and salt contents in all products. It takes a few extra minutes at first but once you know which foods are better choices, it gets much faster.

Between Jean Paré's *Whole Grain Recipes* and *Nature's Cancer-Fighting Foods* by Verne Varona, I found plenty of interesting recipes and choices to reduce the amount of red meat and high starch or processed foods in our diet. I seek out recipe books everywhere I go, using the Internet search engines to add to my collection. I find recipes I like and then try to clean them up as much as I can without ruining them. I substitute any fats for sensible ones by changing butter or canola oil to coconut or olive, white flour to whole grain or brown rice flour, sugar to stevia, honey or maple syrup with sugarless applesauce for bulk. I can make sugar-free cookies that will make your teeth sing, they're so sweet. The secret is pureed figs or dates. I find these tips and pass them on to my friends.

Finding recipes *before* heading to the grocery store will steer you toward making healthier choices at every meal. On the weekends, I often take recipe books or a magazine with recipes in it along on whatever we're doing. I check for anything exciting or new I'd like to try. Each Monday, I make a meal plan for the week

I have recently been loaned a copy of *Eat To Live*, written by Joel Fuhrman, M.D., and sanctioned by the famous Dr. Oz. I would highly recommend this way of eating for anyone needing to lose some serious weight quickly. It is super healthy, filling and sensible but best of all, it is very anti-cancer geared. More veggies, fruits, beans and nuts; less animal products, saturated oils and unfulfilling carbs. It allows you a glass of alcohol a day so my husband is in.

I also delved into Daniel W. Nixon's *Cancer Recovery Eating Plan* because I want to continue to detoxify on occasion. After what I've been through, I was going to do everything I could to make sure I now had a difficult breeding ground for cancer to grow in.

I thoroughly enjoyed the book *Crazy Sexy Cancer Tips* by Kris Carr. This little gem is for every cancer "babe," giving us lots of smiles and suggestions for things like blinging-up a hospital gown, signing up for a patient registry (for your friends to choose gifts from that you might need more than flowers) and a wigilicious section! Think pink! It is complete with recipes and websites you may never have thought of looking for. There's one for rebounders, which I got some great exercises from.

One last book — the *Cancer Vixen* cartoon portrayal of author Marisa Marchetto's ordeal with breast cancer is informative and to the point. It will have you laughing and crying as you recognize your own fang-episodes. Thanks to my thoughtful daughter Karly for brightening my day with that one!

Some of the reading I did on my journey:

Bauman, Edward M., and Helayne L. Waldman. *The Whole-Food Guide for Breast Cancer Survivors: A Nutritional Approach to Preventing Recurrence.* New Harbinger Publications, Inc., 2012.

Campbell, T. Colin, and Thomas M. Campbell. *The China Study: The Most Comprehensive Study of Nutrition Ever Conducted and the Startling Implications for Diet, Weight Loss, and Long-Term Health.* BenBella Books, 2005.

Carr, Kris. *Crazy Sexy Cancer Tips.* Skirt!, 2007.

Dyer, Diana. *A Dietitian's Cancer Story: Information & Inspiration for Recovery & Healing.* Swan Press, 2010.

Fuhrman, Joel. *Eat To Live: The Amazing Nutrient-Rich Program for Fast and Sustained Weight Loss*. Little, Brown and Company, 2012.

Lee, John R., David Zava, and Virginia Hopkins. *What Your Doctor May Not Tell You About Breast Cancer: How Hormone Balance Can Help Save Your Life*. Warner Books, Inc., 2003.

Marchetto, Marisa Acocella. *Cancer Vixen*. Alfred A. Knopf, 2006.

Nixon, Daniel W. *The Cancer Recovery Eating Plan: The Right Foods to Help Fuel Your Recovery*. Random House of Canada Limited, 1994.

Olivotto, Ivo, Karen Gelmon, and Urve Kuusk. *Intelligent Patient Guide to Breast Cancer: All You Need to Know to Take an Active Part in Your Treatment*. Gordon Soules Book Publishers, 2001.

Paré, Jean. *Company's Coming: Whole Grain Recipes*. Company's Coming Publishing Co., 2007.

Spiller, Gene, and Bonnie Bruce. *Cancer Survivor's Nutrition & Health Guide: Eating Well and Getting Better During and After Cancer Treatment*. Prima Lifestyles, 1996.

Stamets, Paul. *Mycelium Running: How Mushrooms Can Help Save the World*. Ten Speed Press, 2005.

Varona, Verne. *Nature's Cancer-Fighting Foods*. Reward Books, 2001.

Walker, Morton. *Jumping For Health: A Guide to Rebounding Aerobics.* Avery Publishing Group, 1989.

Wolfe, David. *Superfoods: The Food and Medicine of the Future.* North Atlantic Books, 2009.

Appendix E

Recommended Websites

A great breast self-examination site:
http://www.checkyourboobies.org

Alcohol and your health:
http://www.health.com/health/article/0,,20410314,00.html

A link for grief:
http://www.cancersurvivors.org/Coping
/end%20term/stages.htm

Army of Women
http://www.armyofwomen.org

Breast Cancer Society of Canada
http://www.bcsc.ca

Canadian Breast Cancer Foundation
http://www.cbcf.org

Canadian Cancer Society
http://www.cancer.ca

Canadian Medical Association
http://www.cma.ca

David Suzuki Foundation
"Dirty Dozen" cosmetic chemicals to avoid:
http://davidsuzuki.org/issues/health/science/toxics
/dirty-dozen-cosmetic-chemicals/

Facing Cancer Together
http://www.facingcancer.ca

For depression:
http://www.depressionhurts.ca

Grass Roots Health
Information about the importance of vitamin D:
http://www.grassrootshealth.net

Sugar Busters Diet Food Lists
http://lowcarbdiets.about.com/od/sugarbusters/a
/sugarbustrlists.htm

Sugar and Cancer: Is There a Connection?
https://www.caring4cancer.com/go/cancer/nutrition
/questions/sugar-and-cancer-is-there-a-connection.htm

Links about sugar consumption:
http://www.sugarstacks.com/blog/

Look Good Feel Better: Helping Women with Cancer
http://www.lgfb.ca

Rethink Breast Cancer: A young women's breast cancer
    organization keeping it pink and cool
    http://rethinkbreastcancer.com/about-rethink/

National Comprehensive Cancer Network (NCCN)
    Staging Guide:
    http://www.nccn.com/understanding-cancer
    /cancer-staging.html

Sunlight, Nutrition and Health Research Center
    http://www.sunarc.org

Susan G. Komen Breast Cancer Foundation
    http://www.komen.org

The Campaign for Safe Cosmetics
    http://www.safecosmetics.org

The taking L-glutamate while receiving chemo debate:
    http://www.livestrong.com/article
    /482174-negatives-of-l-glutamine/

Toxic Effects: Everyday Exposures — strategies for limiting your
    exposure
    http://www.everydayexposures.com

Appendix F

Cancer Highway Travel Tips

1   Your life often depends on your attitude. Are you doing what you can to avoid cancer or are you unconsciously creating the perfect environment to aid cancer growth? Every hour of every day, an average of 21 people will be diagnosed with some type of cancer, and nine people will die from the disease. What makes you think you won't be one of them? It's never too early to start fighting cancer.

2   Be proactive about your health and if necessary, be persistent. Don't let a chronic issue go. If you are not satisfied with a doctor's prognosis, you are entitled to another opinion (although you might have to pay for a private one). Unless you're comatose, never leave your life entirely in someone else's hands. Researching the matter will help. Knowledge is everything.

3   You might get frustrated with the frequent waiting periods between tests. Believe it sometimes or not, the medical staff is there to help and most of them are very overworked. Use honey, not gale-force winds, to get

through this ride. Although if someone is being abusive or unnecessarily difficult, ask to speak to the head nurse or hospital administrator.

Healthy fruit or baked goods, flowers from your garden or a handwritten thank-you note are ALWAYS a great way to back up your appreciation for good, caring service. It also feels nice to make someone else's day a little brighter and helps pave a friendlier path for the next patient.

4 For more information about the different types of breast cancer see this website:
http://www.bcsc.ca/p/41/l/75/t/Breast-Cancer-Society-of-Canada-Types-of-Breast-Cancer

5 Buy a small notebook to carry with you at all times. Record everything from receptionist's names, appointment dates and instructions to be followed. You can request a copy of test results for your own records.

6 If you are in the habit of shaving your legs and/or armpits, buy an electric razor to ensure you do not cut yourself. When you lose sensation in an area due to surgery, it's hard to tell how hard you are pressing with a blade. Don't take chances. And don't use your husband's electric razor without permission. Yours wouldn't be the first marriage to end over unexpected armpit hairs stuck in a razor head.

7 It really helped me to have an inspirational song to lift my spirits when needed. I share one of my favourites, a song by Canadian band Great Big Sea, "Ordinary Day," at the end of this book.

8 The recommended alcoholic consumption for women is no more than one-half to one drink a day (based on 5 ounce glasses of wine or one of any spirit). Once over that, any positive effect alcohol has on your system becomes detrimental. Most men, I'm jealous to say, can handle two a day.

9 Reconstruction is a popular choice and can be done at the same time as a partial or full breast mastectomy (removal). It practically eliminates the risk of future cancer and gets you closer to your former self versus waiting for the mastectomy to heal and then proceeding. Once the skin is radiated, it is less pliable to work with, so pre-radiation recon is recommended.

10 Your spouse or caregiver might be having issues dealing with cancer. Look for support groups in your area or try to link them with someone you know who has been through the experience. Call the Canadian Cancer Society at 1-888-939-3333.

11 Keep moving, even when you don't feel like it. Especially when you don't feel like it. A breath of fresh air does wonders for the mind and body, sending oxygen to your healthy cells and pumping blood in all the right places to speed your recovery. Start by putting one foot in front of the other. Set a goal to walk 10 minutes, then 20, progressing as the days go by.

12 Surround yourself with friends. Don't shut them out. Open that door as wide as you can. Embrace the anonymous saying: "I believe that friends are quiet angels who

sit on our shoulders and lift our wings when we forget
how to fly."

13 Protect yourself from unnecessary cell-damaging toxins.
Read the labels on everything, not only on your food
packages but on your cleaning and beauty products as
well. Try to use natural shampoos, conditioners and hair
dyes without parabens or ammonia, lotions without SLS,
SLES, PG or isopropyl alcohol.

Use natural products with simple ingredients whenever possible.

14 Vitamin E has not been proven to fade scars but it does
promote faster healing. If you are concerned about a new
scar stretching, apply vitamin E before taping the area
tightly with paper tape. Once the scar fades from pink
to white, it has healed.

15 Can't give up the sugar? Give yourself a good scare by
reading this article titled: Ten Studies Showing the Link
Between Sugar and Increased Cancer Risk:

   http://www.naturalnews.com/024827_cancer_
   sugar_women.html

Also check out this other informative website on sugar
and how it affects your insulin levels. It explains how excess insulin may encourage cancer cells to grow. If you
want to know more, follow up on some of the excellent
references listed.

   https://www.caring4cancer.com/go/cancer/
   nutrition/questions/sugar-and-cancer-is-there-a-
   connection.htm

Still giving in to your sweet tooth? Start using sugar
substitutes like stevia, agave syrup, natural honey, pureed

dates or figs, maple syrup, anything but refined sugar, white or brown. Try my Sinless Chocolate Macaroons, recipe included in this book.

16 Talk to a cancer survivor.
Community cancer societies hold meetings where you can sit and chat with other women who are in the process of beating cancer or have come out the other end.

The Canadian Cancer Society has a service called the Cancer Connection where you can call to talk to someone who has gone through whatever it is you are facing. Experienced volunteers sign up as contacts and you are welcome to ask them anything you need to know. It's free, it takes a load off your mind and you might make yourself a new friend right on the spot.

Call the Canadian Cancer Information Service (1-888-939-3333) to learn more.

17 Have a waiting room time distractor. A book of crosswords, Sudoku, your favourite magazines, a new book. The waits will add up so they would be a great time to get something accomplished. Take your knitting. Take up drawing. I am waiting for the Nintendo people to come up with language-learning programs so I can use my DS to take Spanish. Until then, like a dog chasing a ball I'll keep redoing 500 anagrams.

18 Vitamins and supplements give your body extra fighting tools it might not be getting from your diet. Now is the time to start your new anti-cancer regime. My list includes:

▸ Natural Factors women's multivitamin
▸ Natural Factors Hi Potency B Complex

- ► Omega Factors Wild Fish Oil (anchovy and sardine)
- ► Jarrow Formulas Bone-Up (calcium/magnesium supplement)
- ► Vitamin D 2000 IU
- ► Natural Factors Mixed Vitamin E 400 IU to be taken with the following:
    - ▪ Natural Factors Green Tea Extract 300 mg (each capsule is like drinking 30 cups of tea)
- ► And one teaspoon of Trophic Greens Concentrate with antioxidants mixed into water (contains spirulina, kamut juice, goji berry, acai berry and beet juices) to aid an alkaline pH level.

19 If you want to know how to really help someone battling cancer, it's simply being there for them. Listening, consoling when they need it, laughter when they need it, a spare hug; any small gesture that warms their heart. It's about your time.

20 The CCS recommends you stop using the indoor tanning lamps and beds. They say that "tanned skin is damaged skin—it can lead to premature aging and skin cancer."

Use an SPF (sun protection factor) of 15% or higher when going outdoors whether it's cloudy or sunny. For special occasions, use spray-on tanning products, remembering you still need to use an SPF when out in the sun.

I would like to share, compliments of the Canadian band Great Big Sea, my favourite inspirational song, "Ordinary Day," copied with permission.

Ordinary Day
Written by Alan Doyle and Sean McCann

I've got a smile on my face, I've got four walls around me
The sun in the sky, the water surrounds me
I'll win now but sometimes I'll lose
I've been battered, but I'll never bruise, it's not so bad

And I say way-hey-hey, it's just an ordinary day
and it's all your state of mind
At the end of the day, you've just got to say,
it's all right.

Janie sings on the corner, what keeps her from dying?
Let them say what they want, she won't stop trying
She might stumble, if they push her 'round
She might fall, but she'll never lie down

And I say way-hey-hey, it's just an ordinary day
and it's all your state of mind
At the end of the day, you've just got to say,
it's all right.

In this beautiful life, but there's always some sorrow
It's a double-edged knife, but there's always tomorrow
It's up to you now if you sink or swim,
Keep the faith and your ship will come in.
It's not so bad

And I say way-hey-hey, it's just an ordinary day
And it's all your state of mind
At the end of the day, you've just got to say
I say way-hey-hey, it's just an ordinary day
And it's all your state of mind
At the end of the day, you've just got to say
it's alright

'Cause it's alright, it's alright
'Cause I've got a smile on my face and I've got four walls
     around me

Acknowledgments

Getting a book from the first written word to publication is a lot like raising a child. It takes a community.

First and foremost I have to thank my silently supportive spouse who has left me to do "my thing" in the face of dustbuggies (much larger than bunnies) and months of seclusion and slap-dash meals. Some of the book's proceeds will go to hiring a part-time housekeeper so I can continue working on the next three books. It ain't over yet, honey.

I next acknowledge Dr. Sandi Vestvik, whose life-saving thoroughness (that she provides all patients in her care) can never be underrated or overstated. I'm so thankful that you won this one. I finally understand that it doesn't always work that way. You have a seat at our dinner table anytime for the rest of our lives.

To all the physicians and technicians, receptionists, nurses and care providers I shuffled past, my thanks one more time for you being in such a brutal profession as to deal with the sick and downtrodden. This makes you all saints in my book. You too are welcome at our dinner table anytime.

Next, loving appreciation and thanks for my sister and my children: the best fans money can't buy. I appreciate that my family, especially Dad, allowed me to use my interpretation of the past.

My friends and first readers all deserve huge thanks: Carlie, Jane,

Sandi, Kelly, Terry and Terrie, Dorothy, Karen, Jen, Toni, Sheila, Karly, Lorne, Debra and Andrew McAllister (author of the thriller mystery, *Unauthorized Access*).

A large round of applause for the magical work of editor Lynn Shervill who took the sloppy clay creation on a potter's wheel and reshaped it into my exact vision of a book called *Running From Cancer*. Thank you, Lynn. I'm *your* number one fan.

Big thankful hugs to the Canadian band Great Big Sea for permitting use of their super-inspirational song "Ordinary Day." It pulled me up from a very low place.

And a tip of my swim cap to Sue for her abundance of enthusiasm and uplifting song choices for the gang at aqua aerobics.

Sometimes the smallest gestures can make all the difference . . .

In closing, I would like to expand on my choice to donate some of the proceeds of this book to the Bulkley Valley Health Care and Hospital Foundation in Smithers, B.C. Over twenty thousand people, including cancer patients, access the Valley's only hospital, a place without a CT or MRI scanner. Physicians must air vac patients to Vancouver or send on to Terrace for the life-saving tests. With the newly formed foundation, the hope is to compile enough donations to afford more costly yet sorely needed equipment.

CPSIA information can be obtained at www.ICGtesting.com
Printed in the USA
LVOW132140070613

337567LV00002B/41/P